D1457831

Healing Yourself Through
OKIDO YOGA

Healing Yourself Through
OKIDO YOGA

by Masahiro Oki

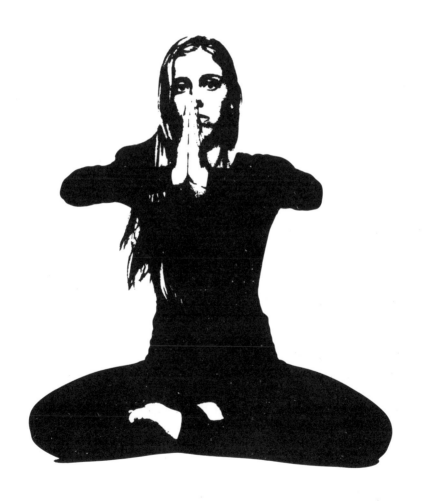

 Japan Publications, Inc.

©in Japan 1977 *by* Masahiro Oki

Photographs by John Fogg
Published by
JAPAN PUBLICATIONS, INC., Tokyo, Japan

Distributed by
JAPAN PUBLICATIONS TRADING COMPANY
200 Clearbrook Road, Elmsford, N.Y. 10523, U.S.A.
1174 Howard Street, San Francisco, Calif. 94103, U.S.A.
P.O. Box 5030 Tokyo International, Tokyo 101–31, Japan

First edition: May, 1977

ISBN 0–87040–380–X
LCCC No. 76–029339

Printed in Japan by Kyodo Printing Co., Ltd.

Preface

Since I began to devote my life to spreading the truth, forty years have passed. Years ago, I realized that Shakyamuni and Gandhi both obtained satori through practicing Yoga. I have devoted myself to applying this ancient form of teaching in modern life. Chronic dis-ease of the mind-body seems to be more and more prevalent in this technological society.

In Japan I have encountered thousands of people whose lifeforce has lost its proper function. As I travelled throughout the world, I began realizing that the problem prevalent in Japan is common to all the nations. Within life in technological society, there exist elements which weaken the innate, natural adaptability. All forms of dis-ease arise in the way people create their life style. Yoga teaches a point of view, "You get what you deserve." One must examine and reevaluate the way he/she lives in order to cultivate the self-healing ability.

More important than healing technique is the teaching of spiritual ways. It is my deep wish that Oriental culture be promoted in Western society to provide the Westerners with spiritual and "religious" mind. As the teachings of the Orient permeate the world, they must undergo modifications and changes suitable for the environment, life style and characteristics of the people in that particular region. However, it is my intention to continue to teach the true Eastern values through Okido Yoga, without oversimplification or distortion. Already the essence of Oriental wisdom has been obscured by changes in its form, as it was geared to the Western understanding.

I began to introduce Okido Yoga in *Practical Yoga*, presenting my understanding of asanas. In *Healing Yourself Through Okido Yoga*, more specifically presented is the Okido way of healing various dis-ease, very common in technological society. What science seems to conclude about the human mind-body and life quality had already been found empirically thousands of years ago in the East. Although many Westerners began to search for an alternative through the findings of the ancient philosophical way of life, the modern people in the East have taken their tradition for granted. Presumably, the West will absorb the ancient Oriental teachings, which will inevitably find its way back to the East as the adverse effects of technological pollution of the mind-body start to prevail there.

I am indebted to my students who devoted themselves to the creation of this book. Shu Uwajima, who structured the book and conducted negotiations with the publisher, is manager of the Okido Yoga Dojo in Boston and Tokyo. Yukiko Iino, who teaches the Taiken Process in New York, has organized my teaching and translated it into English. Currently, she studies under my guidance at the Dojo in Mishima, Japan. In the near future, Ms. Iino will be managing a center for Okido in New York. Anthony Valenti contributed much of his energy and time to writing the first draft of the instruction for Shusei taiso. He has studied with Mr. Uwajima in Boston. Together with Mr. Uwajima, Osamu Tatsumura contributed his first-hand knowledge on Shusei taiso, advising Ms. Iino in the final stage of the book. Mr. Tatsumura has been residing at the Dojo in Mishima for the past several years and assisted me in the individual Shusei sessions, among other countless tasks. Joanna Rotte, a writer for the East and West Journal, who also studies at Mishima currently, assisted in editing. Akemi Hamase, who joined the Dojo after returning from England, helped with proofreading. My special thanks to John Fogg, who photographed the exercises, modelled by Andrea Stronov, who conducts imformal Okido classes in New York.

There are many more; I want to acknowledge all my students, Japanese and Westerners, who render their loyal support and devotion daily in making my work possible.

February, 1977
Mishima, Japan

Masahiro Oki

Contents

A Freely Rendered Collection of Okido Thoughts

The *Shusei Gyoho* described in this book is one of many forms of discipline of Okido Yoga. The exercises prescribed are geared for those living with the strain, tension and maladies resulting from the technological confusion of Western society. Through diligent daily practice of Okido Yoga, it is possible to heighten adaptability to today's environment while re-creating one's self-healing ability.

As a whole, Shusei exercise is a variation of Hatha Yoga with emphasis on *tanden* breathing. Just as the ancient healing arts of acupuncture, shiatsu, yoga and herbalism were empirically derived from an understanding of natural law, Shusei Gyoho is the fruit of my own life-long personal observation and experience. Even now, no scientific explanation has been found for the apparent wonders and esoteric healing effects of Shusei Gyoho. I have assisted tens of thousands of Japanese, Westerners and Africans throughout the world in healing themselves of dis-ease that had been termed incurable by Western and/or Oriental medicine practitioners.

There are varying levels of consciousness in doing exercise. When a person stimulates his body through movement without awareness, it is *Undo* (calisthenics). When an awareness of the physiological interrelationships among, for example, the skeletal structure, muscles and internal organs is added, it becomes *Taiso* (exercise). Shusei—transformation—Taiso operates on this level in that it is conscious exercise to correct postural distortion, skeletal misalignment and improper breathing. From this incipient stage of taiso, a person learns tanden strengthening and proper breathing, thereby progressing to the next level, *Dozen* (dynamic Zen). Dozen is essential to pure, inseparable mind-body discipline. Thus, it is intended through Okido Yoga that a personal, wholistic approach to health be discovered by each participant, while, ever faithful to the law of change, not becoming stuck in any one dogma or belief system. The point is maintaining stability by experiencing what is actual or true.

Together, we are living within infinite harmony maintained by life-force, given by *Kami* (God). Health is the state of balance of all functions of the life-force. As adaptability is cultivated and heightened, it becomes possible to live cooperatively even within our modern technological environment. This ability to adapt I call Nature. Health and Nature are synonymous; actualized, they are satori, the universal ultimate—a condition realized only when the mind-body is pure and the way of life transformed. In satori, a person ultilizes his/her potential to its fullest, and devotes hunself/herself to others willingly, joyfully, productively and gratefully. The spirit of Okido, integrated from experienced application of the true principles of science and philosophy, is the spirit of the religious mind.

Okido Yoga

Okido Yoga is a way of life based on truth derived from experience that integrates science, philosophy and religion. Truth is tested against the three principles of universal law: continuous change, balance maintainance and stability. The culmination is mind-body discipline that seeks utmost stability by utilizing innate balance provided by the life-force (*Kami*) within continuous change.

Okido Yoga has amalgamated practices and teachings of classical Indian Yoga, Yin-Yang philosophy Taoism, Martial Arts and both Oriental and Western medicine, whereby the whole stands more powerful than the sum of its derived parts. Seated in these time-tested truths, Yoga, then, is infinite consciousness, the guiding compass for every moment of life.

It is the intention of Okido to awaken the inner wisdom: physically through Hatha Yoga, socially through Karma Yoga and spiritually through Raja Yoga. These three have inspired the creation of many *gyoho*—discipline in keeping with natural law—by means of which the mind-body is naturally actualized as a full human being. This is the process of elevation to *Busho*, or the innate, essential spirit of every man and woman.

Unlike Western and Oriental medicine which tend to approach disease with a physiological or scientific viewpoint only, Okido Yoga, in its short history, has searched for the truth of life by wholistically examining human spirituality, life quality and mind-body differences manifested in tens of thousands of individuals. Conclusively, the thrust of Okido Yoga is to enable the practitioner to heal and fully realize himself/herself by discipline that adjusts the autonomic nervous system—the (unconscious" regulator of life—and strengthens *tanden*—conscious center of life. Hence, the individual becomes master of his/her own life; that is, achieves *satori*.

Shusei Gyoho

According to Okido Yoga the major causes of all dis-ease are
1) postural distortion and skeletal misalignment
2) improper and/or shallow breathing
3) poor blood quality from an inappropriately balanced diet
4) improper spiritual attitude and way of thinking
Each of these and all together make for an inappropriate life style.

This book is primarily focused upon the first two causes. From studying the exercises, the immediate aim of Shusei gyoho emerges: to eliminate chronic distortion of the mind-body that causes dis-ease. That is because a person must beign somewhere if he/she is to change him/herself; so, begin with taiso.

Meanwhile, the larger and long-range purpose of Shusei gyoho is to enable the individual to activate his/her life-force towards self-healing. Fundamentally, this is accomplished by the taiso in this book which, overall, are designed to eventually induce permanent change in the breathing process. With transformation of breathing comes vitalization of the life-force; with vitalization of the life-force comes wholistic healing and, consequently, a transformed mind-body.

True gyoho is not simply that which adjusts posture or diet, or even cures dis-ease. True gyoho changes life. It recognizes change and makes use of corrective measure to establish appropriate balance and maintain utmost stability. The result of true gyoho is a transformed—natural—life style.

Western and Oriental Medicine Applied to Shusei Gyoho

Both Western and Oriental medicine have points of advantage and points of defect. Okido Yoga combines the advantages and uses them in application to an appropriate situation at the proper time. In Okido Yoga terms that is what is meant by "natural" —cultivated adaptability—way to satori. Improper attitudes, which lead to inappropriate action, which creates dies-ease, do not exist in the state of satori. There is no illness in satori.

Modern western medicine has advanced so called "cures" for various conditions which have come to be signified by various names. In general, these names designate which part of the physiological body is afflicted. This indicates that even though modern medicine is the accumulation of excellent research, its view is partial. At the same time, regarding people, its view is not individualized. In short, it is concerned with symptoms of dis-ease that exist in the same part of many people. Check-ups are given to put a name to the condition in order to prescribe generally, previously established treatment; but a check-up serves only to describe the condition of the moment of the check-up. Such practices, therefore, are invalid.

Traditional Oriental medicine recognizes the constant changes undergone by the mind-body. It has attempted to grasp the dynamic, flowing quality of an individual's life-force, applying different treatment to each person and changing treatment as the condition of dis-ease changes. Of course, unfortunately, today much of Oriental medicine has lost its original intuitive wisdom; in so doing, like unto Western medicine, it limits itself to already specified treatment. For example, this occurs among acupuncturists who treat certain meridians for certain named illnesses, without really considering the energy flow of the whole body.

In truth, the dis-ease of each individual is individual, stemming from a particular whole way of life; so, it requires individual treatment, changing the whole way of life. This is the understanding of Okido Yoga, which has integrated the physiological knowledge of modern Western medicine and the wholistic approach of traditional Oriental medicine. In addition and fundamentally, Okido Yoga means to cultivate self-reliance by bringing forth the ability to self-heal.

Mental Focusing

In each stage of an exercise, try to keep your mind focused on the part of the body which the exercise is meant to stimulate. Simply draw all of your attention to that area as if you were helping to draw all of the healing energy in your body to one point.

Doing this will help you to do the exercise more efficiently because in all yoga practice the energies of the mind are so closely interrelated with those of the breath and body. For example, if your mind is distracted as you do an exercise, you will tend to revert back to a shallow or haphazard form of breathing. When you stop breathing deeply from tanden, you deprive your body of the flexibility and strength which is needed to do the exercise properly.

In other words, when the essential harmony of mind, breath and body is disrupted, the exercise is only partially effective at best. So by controlling your mental energy (keeping it focuses on the part of the body you wish to heal) and by controlling your breath (always breathing deeply and evenly from tanden) you will continue to improve your ability to control the energy of your body. As you continue your practice in this manner, your movements will gradually become steady, smooth and precise.

How to Use This Book

Each Shusei Taiso is effective only if used properly. Approach the exercises one at a time making sure that you first study both the instructions and the photographs carefully in order to form a mental picture of the exercise as a whole. Then try the exercise slowly and carefully several times until you feel comfortable with all phases of it.

You will derive maximum benefit from doing these exercises only if the energies of your mind, breath and body are working together in natural harmony. To allow this harmony to develop takes time and careful, methodic practice. Rushing or pushing yourself excessively beyond your limits will only disrupt the natural process of self-healing.

To simplify your practice, each of the exercises is presented in three step sequence:

Sequence	Breathing Pattern	
Step 1		
The Starting Posture	Breathe normally from tanden—Inhale.	
Step 2		
The Extension	Exhale—Inhale—Retain	Simultaneous
Step 3		
The Corrective Movement	Exhale—Inhale—Relax	

All of the individual movements which make up either the extension (Step 2) or the corrective movement (Step 3) are to be done simultaneously as one movement during a single exhalation, unless otherwise specified.

In the instructions for Step 2 and Step 3 the subordinate movements which make up the total movement are often written separately. However, this is done only for purposes of simplification and in order to emphasize the importance of each of the parts in the total exercise.

Therefore, if you are instructed to arch your back as part of Step 2, you should maintain this arch until you complete the exercise. This will naturally intensify the stimulation and greatly increase the overall effectiveness of the exercise.

Here are some simple guidlines to follow for each of the three steps:

Step 1: Starting Posture

The starting posture is the position from which you will begin an exercise and the position to which you will return in order to relax after completing the exercise. In almost all instances this first step involves minimal exertion. Simply assume the full posture a step at a time as you breathe normally—that is, breathe deeply and evenly from tanden without retaining the breath.

After you are in the starting posture, relax your body briefly. As you take a few more deep breaths, try to become comfortable in this position. Then, inhale and proceed to Step 2.

Step 2: Extension

Step 2 prepares your body for the corrective movement done in Step 3. The stretching movements which make up this part of the exercise creates tension, relaxation, expansion and/or contraction.

Always exhale as you do the extending movements and then inhale and retain your breath for a few seconds; Kumbhaka helps concentrate and strengthen in tanden.

Step 3: Corrective Movement

Shusei Taiso in movement and not in static position achieves a balance to unify all body parts. Yang stimulations are provided for Yin conditions, and vice versa.

After you retain your breath briefly at the conclusion of Step 2, exhale slowly from tanden as you proceed to do the corrective movement in Step 3.

In almost every exercise, you should continue to do the corrective movement for as long as it takes you to complete an exhalation. As you become more adept at doing the movement, strive to prolong both the exhalation and the movement itself. This will intensify the healing effect of the corrective movement, while the slower exhalation and slower movement will also help to strengthen your whole body. Some exercises call for repetitive up-and-down motion of the legs. In practicing such exercises, exhale as you raise the legs, and inhale while bringing them down.

As you practice a particular exercise from day to day, gradually try to increase the number of times you repeat the corrective movement, aiming over a period of time for ten to fifteen repetitions. However, always go slowly and carefully at your own pace. A few repetitions of an exercise done with care will be much more effective than several done hastily and improperly.

You may want to practice the subordinate movements separately at first and then proceed to combine each of them until you gradually acquire a feeling for the form of the movement as a whole. However, always strive toward doing all of the separate parts of Step 2 or Step 3 as one smooth action with all the parts of your body working in unison.

With practice, this kind of total body action will come easily and naturally.

In the text for Step 2 the instructions occurring most frequently are "Pull the chin in" and "Stretch the Achilles tendons." Both of these extending movements are simple centering techniques which help to stimulate the tanden region, to name but only few effects.

"Pull the chin in" extends the back of the neck and the rest of the spine in the direction of the head away from tanden. Therefore, the chin should be pulled down toward the chest without bending the neck. This is the same technique employed in the *seiza meiso* posture.

"Stretch the Achilles' tendons" extends the backs of the ankles and of the legs (hemstring muscles) away from tanden. If you are lying on your back, this motion will cause your toes to point upto the ceiling; your heels may slightly raise off the floor.

These two opposing tensions are balanced in tanden, giving the body a stabilizing center of energy. Consequently, it becomes easier and more natural to breath deeply and evenly from this energy source as you do each of the exercises.

A simple but effective centering exercise is to practice these two movements by themselves while lying in a prone position. First, inhale, then pull the chin in, and stretch the Achilles tendons as you exhale. Concentrate on breathing deeply from tanden. This exercise will greatly improve your ability to regulate your breathing and will also strengthen tanden and help to rid your mind-body of tension.

Resting After Each Exercise

Shusei Taiso produces a deep, powerful healing effect. Quite often stimulation is concentrated in parts of the body which have been chronically stiff, inactive or misaligned. Consequently, resting after each exercise, thus allowing your body time to adjust to the internal changes induced by the exercise, is an absolute necessity.

After you have finished the corrective movement, refrain from relaxing into a random posture without any attention to your breathing. After Step 3, you should inhale, as you return to the starting posture. Remain in the starting posture briefly. Rest your whole body as you continue to breathe deeply from tanden in a slow, relaxed manner.

While you are resting, continue to focus your mind on the part of your body which has just been stimulated. Simply draw your attention to that part of the body, in order to fully experience the effect of the exercise.

When you feel fully rested, repeat the exercise. The amount of time you should spend resting in between exercises will, of course, vary from day to day depending on your condition—as will the number of repetitions of each exercise that you choose to do. Simply use your won good judgment. Remain sensitive to the changing needs of your own body.

Always keep in mind that taking the time to rest and breathe deeply after you do an exercise is as important a part of self-healing as the exercise itself.

Shusei Taiso

Spinal Stimulation

The spinal column is the body's longitudinal axis designed to insure proper distribution of body weight. Spinal misalignment can be attributed to weight strain, habitual misuse of the body and dis-ease. Distortion is actually one of the body's means of protection. Since each vertebra corresponds to particular internal organs and the operation of the nervous system, spinal misalignment reveals internal malfunction. The scientific explanation for this is that the autonomic nerves, which regulate the internal organs, originate at the base of the brain and travel the length of the spinal column. Thus, the neck, standing as the communicative path from the brain to the internal organs, is vital to life. In the Japanese language, death at an early age is called *yosetsu*, or "distorted neck."

Actually, the whole interrelationship is circular. Spinal misalignment affects the spinal nerves, which originate in the vertebral canals. Irritated spinal nerves, in turn, give birth to various physiological problems. In the other direction, physiological problems irritate the spinal nerves, giving birth to spinal misalignment.

Because spinal distortion as a protective device actually serves to maintain the Yin-Yang balance within the body, mere adjustment of the spine can be dangerous. However, specific exercise, consciously selected to give appropriate Yin or Yang stimulation, is a proper means to gradual correction. Such exercise also strengthens the spinal muscles, connective tissue, internal organs and, most importantly, develops tanden—central to healthy operation of the mind-body.

17

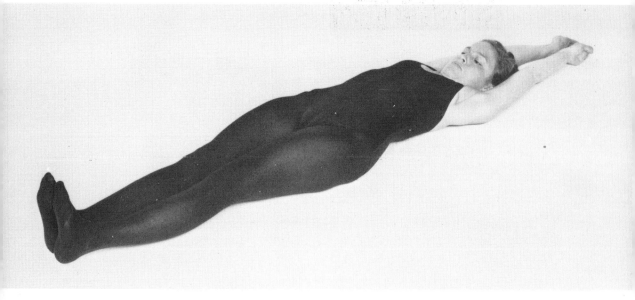

EXERCISE 1   **Cervical 1 and 2**

Starting Posture

Normal Breathing

Lie on the back, with legs extended, and feet together.

Extend the arms alongside the head with the backs of the hands touching. Make loose fists.

Relax in this posture briefly, then inhale.

Extension

Exhaling

Pull the chin in. Tighten the fists and stretch the arms without raising them off the floor. Stretching the Achilles tendons, raise the heels about three inches.

Inhale deeply, then, retain the breath while holding this posture for a few seconds.

Corrective Movement

Exhaling

Now move the legs up and down slowly without bending the knees.

(Keeping the fists tight, continue to stretch the arms as you raise and lower the legs.)

Inhale, return to the starting posture and relax.

Note

The raising and lowering of the legs in this exercise are repeated in corrective movement of exercises 1 through 6.

As you do this movement, remember these points:

1) Keep the chin in without lifting the back of the head off the floor.

2) Keep the Achilles tendons stretched.

3) Raise the heels no higher than six to eight inches off the floor.

4) Do not let the heels touch the floor as you lower the legs.

5) It is especially important, in most of corrective movements done in step 3 of Okido exercises, to continue the movement during exhalation.

EXERCISE 2   **Cervical 3**

Starting Posture

Normal Breathing

Lie on the back, legs extended and feet spread a few inches apart. Turn the feet inwards so that the big toes are touching and then spread the heels further apart.

Extend the arms alongside the head, palms up, and spread the hands about six inches apart.

Relax in this posture briefly, then, inhale.

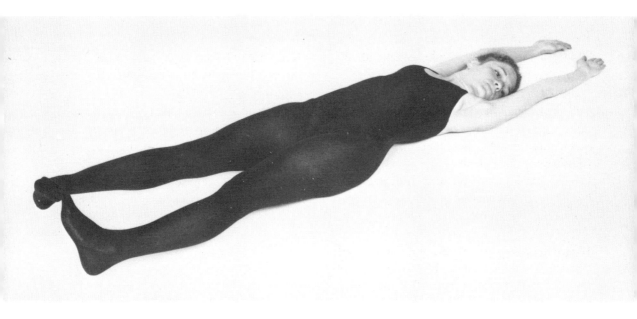

Extension

Exhaling

Pull the chin in. Stretch the arms without raising them off the floor.

Stretching the Achilles tendons, raise the heels about three inches.

Inhale deeply, then, retain the breath while holding this posture for a few seconds.

Corrective Movement

Exhaling

Keeping the toes together and heels apart, move the legs up and down without bending the knees—as in exercise 1.

As you move the legs, slowly turn the head from side to side keeping the chin in. Continue to stretch the arms upwards.

(Turn the neck from side to side with a slow stretching motion, taking care not to let the head drop to the floor).

Inhale, return to the starting posture and relax.

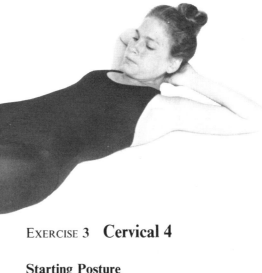

EXERCISE 3 **Cervical 4**

Starting Posture

Normal Breathing

Lie on the back, legs extended, and feet together.

Clasp the hands behind the head just above the neck, and rest the elbows on the floor. Relax in this posture briefly, then, inhale.

Extension

Exhaling

Pull the chin in. Keeping the elbows on the floor, stretch them out to the sides.
Stretching the Achilles tendons, raise the heels about three inches.
Inhale, holding this posture and retain the breath for a few seconds.

Corrective Movement

Exhaling

Keeping the elbows on the floor and hands clasped behind the neck, raise the head off the floor as high as possible, meanwhile continuing to stretch the elbows out.
At the same time, slowly move the legs up and down without bending the knees—as in exercise 1.
(The shoulder blades should not rise off the floor, but the neck should be stretched as much as possible while keeping the chin in.)
Inhale, return to the starting posture and relax.

EXERCISE **4** **Cervical 5**

Starting Posture

Normal Breathing

Lie on the back, legs extended, and spread the feet waist-width apart.
Clasp the hands together behind the head just above the neck, and rest the elbows on the floor.
Relax in this posture briefly, then, inhale.

Extension

Exhaling

Pull the chin in. Keeping the elbows on the floor, stretch them out to the sides.
Stretching the Achilles tendons, raise the heels about three inches.
Inhale deeply, then, retain the breath while holding this posture for a few seconds.

Corrective Movement

Exhaling

Keeping the feet together, move the legs up and down without bending the knees as in exercise 1.
(Continue to stretch the elbows out to the sides as you raise and lower the legs.)
Inhale, return to the starting posture and relax.
See photo in exercise 3, for the positions of the arms, neck and head. In exercise 4, the chest is arched and legs are spread.

EXERCISE **5** **Cervical 6**

Starting Posture

Normal Breathing

Lie on the back, with legs extended, and feet together.
Make the arms 'L' shaped, fingers pointing in the direction of the head, elbows on the floor.
Relax in this posture briefly, then, inhale.

Extension

Exhaling

Pull the chin in. Tighten the fists. Stretch the elbows out to the sides.
Stretching the Achilles tendons, raise the heels about three inches.
Inhale, holding this posture and retain the breath for a few seconds.

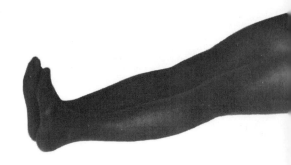

Corrective Movement
Exhaling
Press down on the floor with the fists and elbows; and keeping the feet together, move the legs up and down without bending the knees—as in exercise 1.
Inhale, and return to the starting posture and relax.

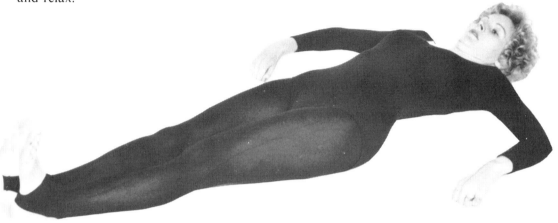

EXERCISE **6 Cervical 7**

The starting posture and sequence of movements in this exercise are basically the same as in exercise 5, the only difference being in the position of the arms.
In extension, however, bend the elbows towards the feet.

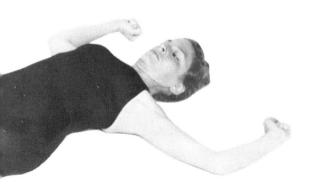

EXERCISE **7 Thoracic 1**

Starting Posture
Normal Breathing
Lie on the back, legs extended, and feet spread waist-width apart.
With palms up, place the fingertips on the chin. Rest the elbows on the floor.
Extension
Exhaling
Pull the chin in. Stretch the Achilles tendons. Keeping the elbows on the floor and the fingertips firmly on the chin, stretch the arms out to the sides.
Inhale, deeply then, retain the breath while holding this posture for a few seconds.
Corrective Movement
Exhaling
Raise the head and neck off the floor as far as possible, keeping the chin in.
After you finish exhaling, hold this posture and retain the breath for a few seconds. Then, inhale, return to the starting posture and relax.

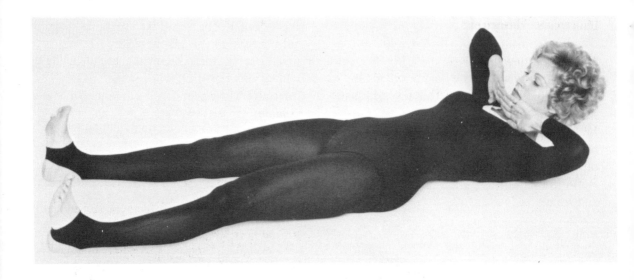

EXERCISE 8   **Thoracic 2**

Starting Posture

Normal Breathing

Lie on the back, the legs extended, and feet spread waist-width apart.

Clasp the hands together behind the neck, and rest the elbows on the floor.

Relax in this posture briefly, then, inhale.

Extension

Exhaling

Pull the chin in. Stretch the Achilles tendons. Bring the elbows together in front of the face.

Inhale deeply, then, retain the breath while holding this posture for a few seconds.

Corrective Movement

Exhaling

Pressing the elbows together rightly, pull the head and neck off the floor, as you continue to hold the chin in.

While pulling the head and neck upwards, take care not to pull the shoulder blades off the floor as well.

After you finish exhaling, hold this posture and retain the breath for a few seconds. Then, inhale, return to the starting posture and relax.

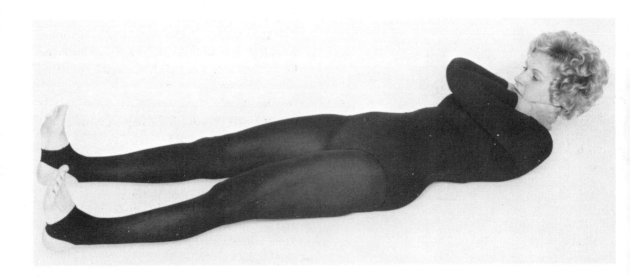

EXERCISE 9 **Thoracic 3**

Starting Posture
Normal Breathing
Lie on the back, legs extended, and feet spread waist-width apart.
Make fists and place them at the sides of the body just below the arm pits. Rest the elbows on the floor.
Relax in this posture briefly, then, inhale.
Extension
Exhaling
Pull the chin in. Stretch the Achilles tendons.
Keeping the arms on the floor, stretch the

elbows out to the sides. At the same time, pull the fists up toward the head.
Inhale deeply, then, retain the breath while holding this posture for a few seconds.
Corrective Movement
Exhaling
Pull the head and neck off the floor while continuing to hold the chin in.
At the same time, arch the lower back off the floor as much as possible so that the chest may be off the floor.
After you finish exhaling, hold this posture and retain the breath for a few seconds. Then, inhale, return to the starting posture and relax.

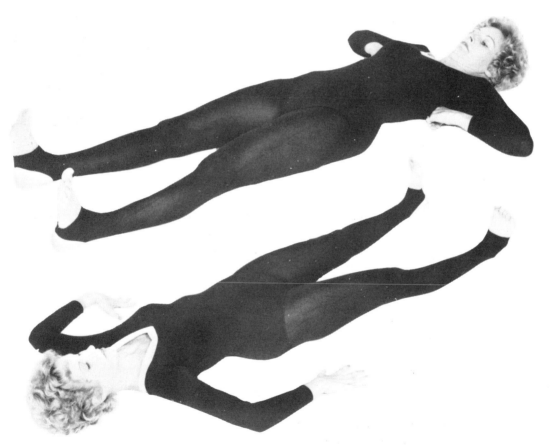

EXERCISE 10 **Thoracic 4**

Starting Posture
Normal Breathing
Lie on the back, legs extended and feet

spread waist-width apart.

Make the arms 'L' shaped, fingers pointing towards the feet, elbows on the floor.

Relax in this posture briefly, then, inhale.

Extension

Exhaling

Pull the chin in. Stretch the Achilles tendons.

Inhale deeply, then, retain the breath while holding this posture for a few seconds.

Corrective Movement

Exhaling

Keeping the head, arms and hands on the floor, pull the arms upwards toward the head. Put pressure on the area of the shoulder blades. Keep the chin down and the Achilles tendons stretched throughout the exhalation.

After exhaling, hold this posture and retain the breath for a few seconds. Then, inhale, return to the starting posture and relax.

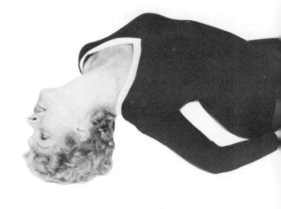

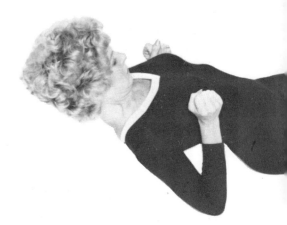

EXERCISE 11   Thoracic 5

Starting Posture

Normal Breathing

Lie on the back, legs extended, and feet together.

Put the hands on the sides of the thighs.

Relax in this posture briefly then inhale.

Extension

Exhaling

Stretch the Achilles tendons. Press down firmly on the floor with the elbows.

Inhale deeply then retain the breath while holding this posture for a few seconds.

Corrective Movement

Exhaling

Keeping the legs, buttocks and elbows on the floor, arch the upper back as high as possible, raising up on the top of the head.

(As you arch upwards, keep the elbows in place, press the hands firmly against the thighs. Continue to stretch the Achilles tendons.)

After you finish exhaling, hold this posture and retain the breath for a few seconds. Then, inhale, return to the starting posture and relax.

Refer to Variation on Fish Pose. (See *Practical Yoga* by the same author, p. 66).

EXERCISE 12   Thoracic 6

Starting Posture

Normal Breathing

Lie on the back, legs extended, feet together, and arms along the side.

Bend the elbows so that the hands are pointing towards the ceiling. Make fists.

Relax in this posture briefly, then, inhale.

EXERCISE 13   Thoracic 7

Starting Posture

Normal Breathing

Sit on the floor between the heels. Reach back and grasp the ankles.

Now, slowly lean back until the head and back are resting flat on the floor—(or lean back as far as possible).

Relax in this posture briefly, then, inhale.

Extension

Exhaling

Pull the chin in. Pull upward on the ankles, bending the elbows only slightly.

Inhale deeply, then, retain the breath while holding this posture for a few seconds.

Corrective Movement

Exhaling

Sit up as for as possible using tanden strength. Keeping the arms close to the body and the chin down to the chest.

(Try to avoid using the elbows for support while sitting up).

After you finish exhaling, hold this posture and retain the breath for a few seconds. Then, inhale, return to the starting posture and relax.

Extension

Exhaling

Stretch the Achilles tendons. Press down firmly on the floor with the elbows. Arch the upper back off the floor, raising up on the top of the head.

Inhale deeply, then retain the breath while holding this posture for a few seconds.

Corrective Movement

Exhaling

From this arched posture, slowly raise the head and neck off the floor until the chin is pressing down firmly on the chest.

At the same time, raise the feet about three inches, stretching the Achilles tendons.

(Try to keep the back arched as you do this part of the exercise.)

After you finish exhaling, hold this posture and retain the breath for a few seconds. Then, inhale, return to the starting posture and relax.

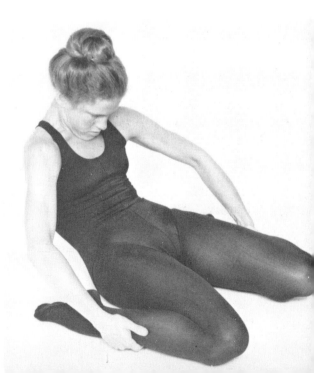

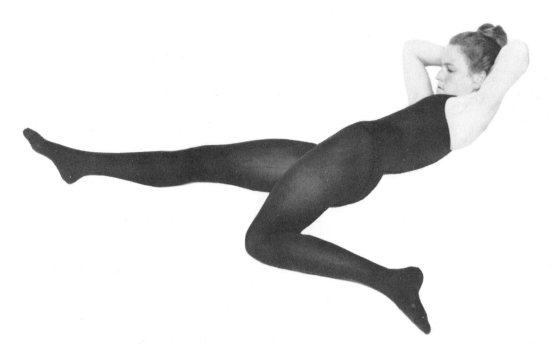

EXERCISE 14   **Thoracic 8**

Starting posture and extension of this exercise are the same as in exercise 13.

Corrective Movement

Exhaling

Raise up on the head, arching the back and buttocks off the floor.

Concentrate on using tanden strength.

After you finish exhaling, hold this posture and retain the breath for a few seconds. Then, inhale, return to the starting posture and relax.

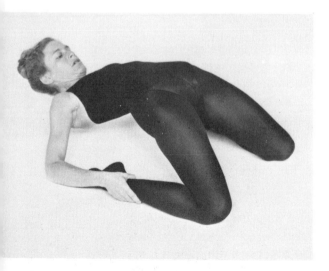

EXERCISE 15   **Thoracic 9**

Starting Posture

Normal Breathing

Lie on the back with the left leg bent at the knee and the right leg stretched out straight. Clasp the hands behind the head just above the neck, and rest the elbows on the floor. Relax in this posture briefly, then, inhale.

Extension

Exhaling

Keeping the elbows on the floor, stretch them out to the sides.

Pull the chin in. Press the left knee down to the floor. Stretch the Achilles tendon in the right leg.

Inhale deeply, then, retain the breath while holding this posture for a few seconds.

Corrective Movement

Exhaling

Stretch the elbows upwards toward the head. Sit up as far as possible, pulling the chin.

After you finish exhaling, hold this posture and retain the breath for a few seconds. Then, inhale, return to the starting posture and relax.

Repeat the exercise with the opposite leg bent. Do the exercise more in the posture which is more difficult for you.

EXERCISE 16 **Thoracic 10**

Starting Posture
Normal Breathing
Sit on the floor with legs extended and feet spread apart one and a half times waist-width.
Extend the arms in front at shoulder level.
Interlock the fingers and turn the palms outwards.
Relax in this posture briefly, then, inhale.

Extension
Exhaling
Pull the chin in, Stretch the Achilles tendons.
Lean back at about 45 degrees and stretch the arms forward.

Corrective Movement
Exhaling
Maintaining this posture, slowly move the head and arms as far as possible from right to left while keeping the arms at shoulder level and the eyes focused on the hands.
Inhale, return to the starting posture and relax.

A

B

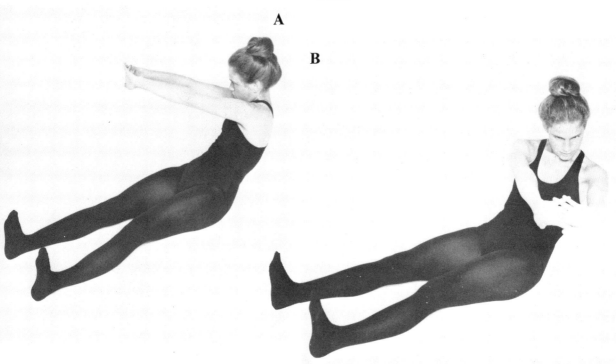

EXERCISE 17 **Thoracic 11**

Starting Posture
Normal Breathing
Lie on the back with the left leg extended and the right leg bent back at the knee.
Grasp the right ankle with the right hand.
Extend the left arm straight up over head, and press against the ear.
Relax in this posture briefly, then, inhale.

Extension
Exhaling
Pull the chin in. Stretch the left Achilles tendon.
Stretch the left arm upwards and press the right knee down to the floor.
Inhale deeply, then, retain the breath while holding this posture for a few seconds.

Corrective Movement

Exhaling

Maintaining this posture, sit up as far as possible while exhaling.

After you finish exhaling, hold this posture and retain the breath for a few seconds. Then, inhale, return to the starting posture and relax.

Repeat the exercise, reversing the positions of the arms and legs. Do the exercise more in the posture which is more difficult.

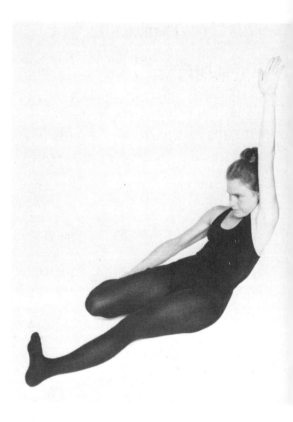

EXERCISE **18**   **Thoracic 12**

Starting Posture

Normal Breathing

Lie on the back, legs extended and feet together.

Extend the arms straight out to the sides, palms down.

Relax in this posture briefly, then, inhale.

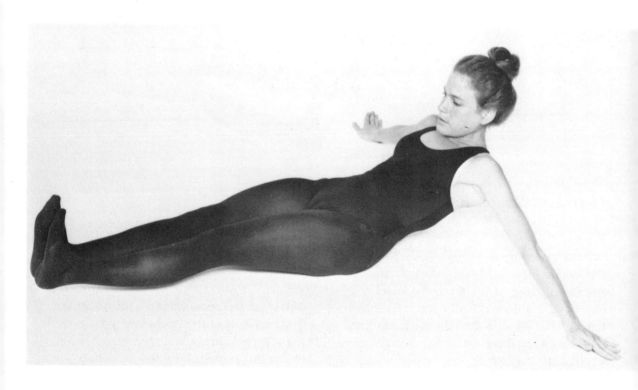

Extension

Exhaling

Pull the chin in. Stretch the Achilles tendons.
Raise the heels two or three inches.
Inhale deeply, then, retain the breath while
holding this posture for a few seconds.

Corrective Movement

Exhaling

Keeping the chin in and sit up to a position
45 degrees from the floor.
(While sitting up, keep the hands firmly on
the floor in the same position as in the starting posture—and avoid bending the elbows.)
After you finish exhaling, hold this posture
and retain the breath for a few seconds.
Then, inhale, return to the starting posture
and relax.

Starting Posture

Normal Breathing

Lie on the back, legs extended and feet
spread apart double the waist-width.
Extend the arms straight out to the sides,
palms down.
Relax in this posture briefly, then, inhale.

Extension

Exhaling

Pull the chin in. Stretch the Achilles tendons.
Stretch the arms out to the sides.
Inhale deeply, then, retain the breath while
holding this posture for a few seconds.

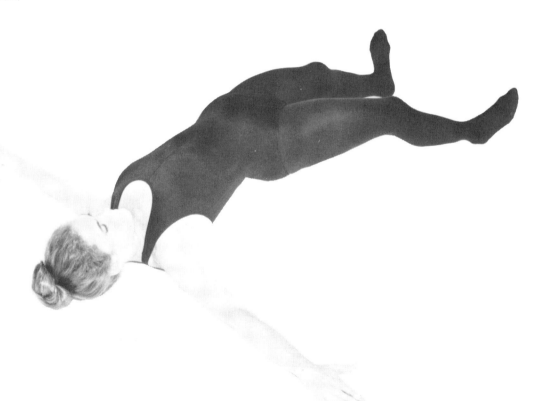

Corrective Movement

Exhaling

Keeping the arms and legs as straight as
possible, press down on the floor with the
heels and hands.
Raise the lower back and buttocks off the
floor as high as possible.

After you finish exhaling, hold this posture
and retain the breath for a few seconds.
Then, inhale, return to the starting posture
and relax.

EXERCISE 20 **Lumbar 2**

Starting Posture
Normal Breathing

Lie on the back, legs extended and feet spread apart as widely as possible.

Extend one arm straight out on the floor directly overhead, with the palm facing inward.

Raise the opposite arm towards the ceiling with the palm facing inward.

Relax in this posture briefly, then, inhale.

Extension
Exhaling

Pull the chin in. Stretch the Achilles tendons and both arms.

Inhale deeply, then, retain the breath while holding this posture for a few seconds.

Corrective Movement
Exhaling

Sit up as far as possible.

After you finish exhaling, hold this posture and retain the breath for a few seconds. Then inhale, return to the starting posture and relax.

Repeat the exercise reversing the positions of the arms, and do more in the posture more difficult.

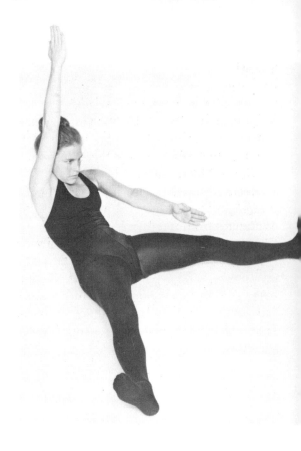

EXERCISE 21 **Lumbar 3**

Starting Posture
Normal Breathing

Lie on the back, legs extended and feet spread apart as widely as possible.

Clasp the hands together behind the head just above the neck and rest the elbows on the floor.

Relax in this posture briefly, then, inhale.

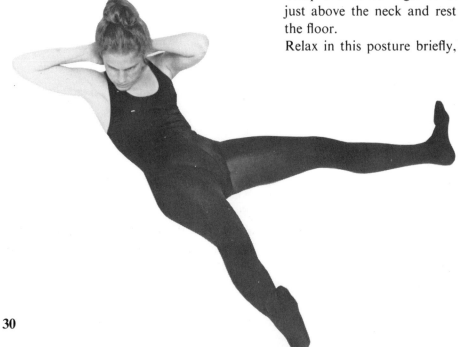

Extension

Exhaling

Pull the chin in. Stretch the Achilles tendons. Keeping the elbows on the floor, stretch them out to the sides.

Inhale deeply, then, retain the breath while holding this posture for a few seconds.

Corrective Movement

Exhaling

Without moving the legs, raise the torso off the floor as follows:

1) Sit straight up to a position about 45 degrees from the floor.

2) At this point continue to sit up as you turn the head and torso as far as possible to one side. (Start to turn at 45 degrees and complete the turn at 90 degrees.)

After you finish exhaling, hold this posture and retain the breath for a few seconds. Then, inhale, return to the starting posture and relax.

Repeat the exercise, turning to the opposite side.

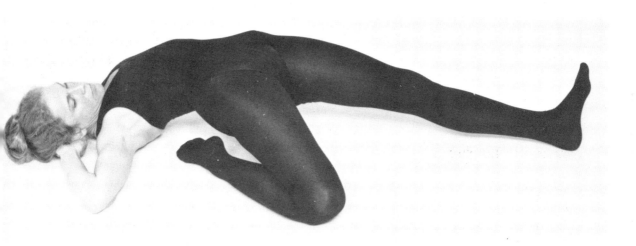

EXERCISE **22** **Lumbar 4**

Starting Posture

Normal Breathing

Lie on the back with the left leg extended and the right leg bent back at the knee. (Do not sit on the heel, but place it close to the side of the hip.)

Clasp the hands behind the head just above the neck and rest the elbows on the floor.

Relax in this posture briefly, then, inhale.

Extension

Exhaling

Pull the chin in. Stretch the Achilles tendons in the outstretched leg.

Keeping the elbows on the floor, stretch them out to the sides.

Raise the buttocks and the lower back off the floor as high as possible.

Inhale deeply, then, retain the breath while holding this posture for a few seconds.

Corrective Movement

Exhaling

Keeping the head, elbows and shoulder blades on the floor, turn the head and upper torso as far as possible from side to side.

(Keep the hips upwards and as stationary as possible.)

Inhale, return to the starting posture and relax.

Repeat the exercise, reversing the positions of the legs. Do more in the posture more difficult for you.

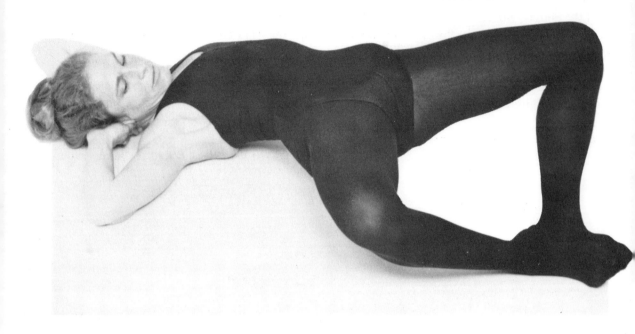

EXERCISE 23   **Lumbar 5**

Starting Posture
Normal Breathing

Lying on the back, join the soles of the feet together and bring them up close to the buttocks.

Clasp the hands behind the head just above the neck and rest the elbows on the floor.

Relax in this posture briefly, then, inhale.

Extension
Exhaling

Pull the chin in.

Keeping the elbows on the floor, stretch them out to the sides.

Raise the buttocks and the lower back off the floor as much as possible, and spreading the knees out to the sides.

Inhale deeply, then, retain the breath while holding this posture for a few seconds.

Corrective Movement
Exhaling

Turn the head and upper body from side to side as in exercise 22.

(Be sure to keep the hips arched upwards and the knees spread apart as you turn from side to side.)

Inhale, return to the starting posture and relax.

Headache

One theory attributes headache to tightening of the blood vessels in the brain; still, medical science has not resolved headache. Whether physiological or psychological in origin, the cause of headache cannot be remedied by drugs.

Simple headache is often an incipient symptom of any one of a number of dis-eases. For example, the most dangerous kind stems from brain dis-ease, such as meningitis, syphilis or tumor. In the case of tumor, it is usually accompanied by persistent, severe headache and nausea without fever. When discovered early on, brain tumor is symptomatically treated by surgical removal.

The most common cause of headache is physiological distortion, such as cervical misalignment and contraction of the base of the skull into the neck. These, as well as intestinal deposits of feces and excessive protein and salt, cause poor pulsing ability of the blood vessels in the brain. The result is blood congestion in the brain—a mind in confusion.

When the muscles of the neck, shoulders and arms become hard, blood circulation to the brain becomes poor; hence, brain cells contract from lack of oxygen, press against the nerves and cause headache. Posture must be corrected to release the muscles, and habitual thoracic breathing must be changed to deep, tanden breathing by means of exercise.

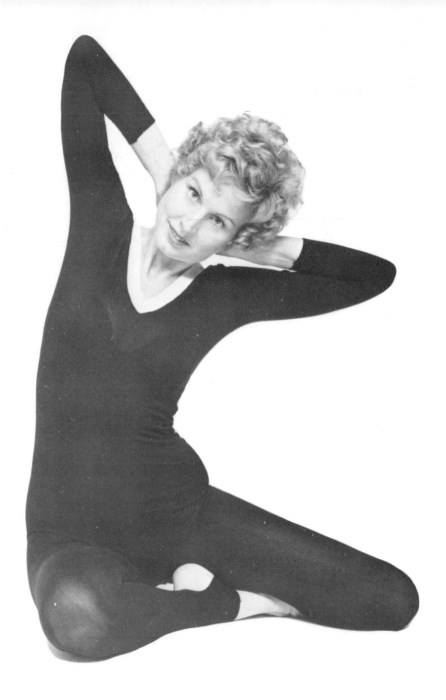

EXERCISE 24 Headache 1

Starting Posture
Normal Breathing

Sit on floor, legs, extended, and feet together. Bend one leg back and out to the side, keeping the knee on the floor and placing the foot next to the hip.

Bend the other leg, placing the foot on the inside thigh of the opposite leg. Keep this knee on the floor also.

(One leg is bent to the outside; the other is bent to the inside.)

Place the hands one on top of the other, behind the head just above the neck.

Relax in this posture briefly, then, inhale.

Extension

Exhaling

Pull the chin in. Press the knees down to the floor. Stretch the elbows up and out to the sides, expanding the ribcage.

Inhale deeply, then, retain the breath while holding this posture for a few seconds.

Corrective Movement

Exhaling

Apply firm pressure to the back of the head with the heels of the hands while bending to one side. Stretch the opposite side of the neck, arm, and upper torso. Try to touch the elbow to the floor.

Inhale, return to center. Exhaling, stretch down to the opposite side. (Do not raise the hips off the floor. Keep the knees in place, chin down, and elbows stretched back.)

Inhale, return to center and relax.

Repeat the exercise alternating the position of the legs. Do the exercise more in the posture more difficult for you.

EXERCISE **25** **Headache 2**

Starting Posture

Normal Breathing

Kneel down with the knees together and arms at the sides. Lower the hips, and sit between the feet.

Place the hands, one on top of the other, behind the head just above the neck.

Relax in this posture briefly, then, inhale.

Extension

Exhaling

Bring the elbows together, pulling the chin in.

Stretch the elbows up, straightening the back. Inhale deeply, then, retain the breath while holding this posture for a few seconds.

Corrective Movement

Exhaling

Press the elbows together, pull firmly on the back of the head, stretch the back of the

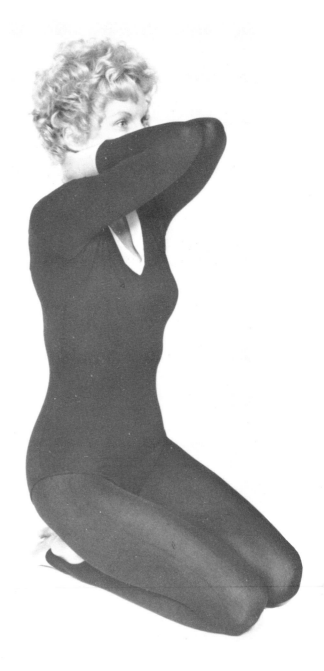

neck up and forward until the chin is pressing down firmly on the chest.

(During this movement, allow the hips to raise slightly off the floor—but not more than two or three inches.)

After you finish exhaling, hold this posture and retain the breath for a few seconds. Inhale, return to the starting posture and relax.

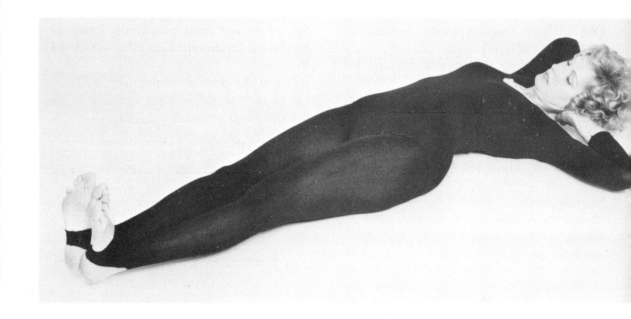

EXERCISE 26　**Headache 3**

Starting Posture

Normal Breathing

Lie on the back, legs extended and feet together.

Place the hands, one on top of the other, behind the head, just above the neck. Rest the elbows on the floor.

Relax in this posture briefly, then, inhale.

Extension

Exhaling

Pull the chin in. Stretch the elbows out to the sides. and Stretch the Achilles tendons. Inhale deeply, and retain the breath while holding this posture for a few seconds.

Corrective Movement

Exhaling

Apply firm pressure to the back of the head with the heels of the hands, while slowly bending to one side, stretching the neck, arm and the upper torso of the other side. (While doing this movement, keep the head and arms on the floor, avoid moving from the waist down.)

Inhale, returning to center.

Exhaling, bend to the opposite side.

Inhale, return to center and relax.

EXERCISE 27　**Headache 4**

Starting Posture

Normal Breathing

Lie on the back, legs extended, and spread the feet apart one and a half times the waist-width.

Place the feet on the floor paralleled to each other.

Join the hands together in prayer fashion (Gasho) about six inches in front of the face, fingertips at eye level, elbows at shoulder level.

Relax in this posture briefly, then, inhale.

Extension

Exhaling

Arch up on the top of the head, lifting the whole torso off the floor.

(At this point, only the feet and the top of the head should be on the floor.)

Keeping the knees apart, press the hands together firmly.

Inhale deeply, then, retain the breath while holding this posture for a few seconds.

Corrective Movement

Exhaling

Slowly move the hips from side to side as far as possible.

(While doing this movement, concentrate on moving the hips.)
Inhale, return to the starting posture and relax.

EXERCISE 28 Headache 5

Starting Posture
Normal Breathing
Lie on the stomach, forehead on the floor, and legs extended.

Spread the feet apart waist-width. Place the hands, one on the top of the other behind the the floor.
Relax in the posture briefly, then, inhale.
Lie on the stomach with the forehead on the floor and legs extended.
Spread the feet apart waist width. Place the hands, one on the of the other behind the head just above your neck. Rest elbows on the floor.
Relax in the posture briefly then inhale.
Extension
Exhaling
Stretch the elbows out to the sides. Lift the

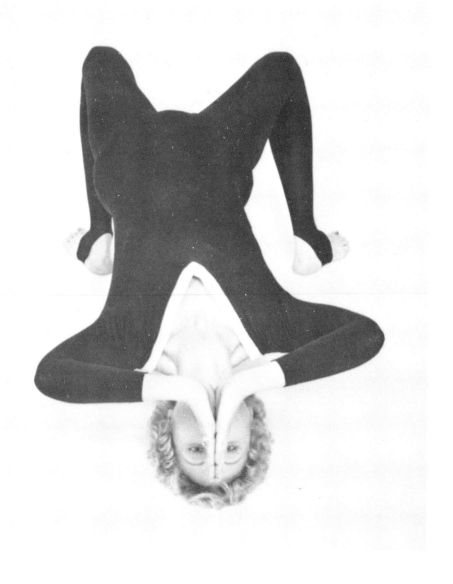

elbows and head about two inches off the floor.

Stretch the Achilles tendons and raise the feet about two or three inches off the floor.

Inhale deeply, retain the breath while holding this posture for a few seconds.

Corrective Movement

Exhaling

Apply firm pressure to the back of the head with the heels of the hands. Bend to one side, slowly stretching the neck, arms and upper torso of the other side—as in exercises 24 and 26.

(Keep the forehead and elbows close to the floor.

Keep the feet off the floor without bending the knees.)

Inhale, returning to center. Exhale, stretch down to the opposite side.

Each time after you finish exhaling, hold the posture and retain the breath for a few seconds before inhaling and returning to the starting posture.

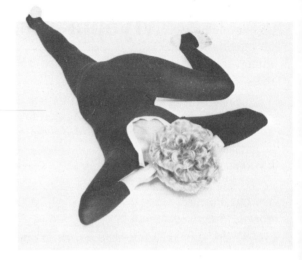

EXERCISE **29   Headache 6**

Starting Posture

Normal Breathing

Lie on the stomach, legs extended, feet together, and forehead on the floor.

Place the hands, one on top of the other, behind the head just above the neck and rest the elbows on the floor.

Keeping the leg on the floor, bend one knee up toward the head and spread the other leg as far as possible.

Relax in this posture briefly, then, inhale.

Extension

Exhaling

Stretching the elbows out to the sides, raise the head and arms off the floor as much as possible.

Pull the chin in. Stretch the Achilles tendons. Inhale deeply, then, retain the breath while holding this posture for a few seconds.

Corrective Movement

Exhaling

Keeping the head and arms raised off the floor, bend to one side. Stretch the neck and the upper torso of the other side. Pull the bent knee toward the head.

Inhale, return to the starting posture and relax.

Repeart the exercise reversing the positions of the legs. Do more in the posture more difficult.

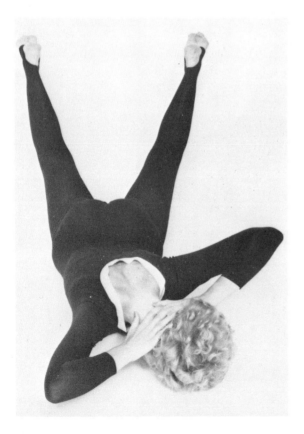

Myopia and Other Vision Problems

The methods for correcting myopia and other vision problems are the same, excepting that for hypermetropia, care must be taken to prevent degeneration from aging. Contraction and hardening of the eyeballs and ciliary and related muscles cause blood congestion and shape distortion. These symptoms stem from chronically distorted posture, mind tension and inappropriate diet—likewise the causes of other dis-ease. It, therefore, occurs that while healing chronic illness of, for example, the kidneys eyesight is simultaneously improved. It follows that to heal eye problems, consider not only the eyes in treatment.

Gyoho is necessary to loosen blood congestion and refraction. Fasting, which eliminates old deposits in the muscles and blood vessels surrounding the eyes, thus relaxing the muscles, is recommended. Conscious blinking, eye exercise (moving the eyes up and down, sideways and circularly), and cold water eye-baths are effective. Asanas such as the arch, headstand and plough poses are helpful, as well as twisting and stretching of the arms and wrists, legs and ankles and torso in all directions.

To relieve stabismus (crossed-eyes), correct distortion of the cervical vertebrae, slackening of the scalp, and unevenness of the scapulae. For astigmatism, inequality of shoulder height and arm power should be balanced.

Within all the physiological approaches to correction, there is one common necessity: to relax the mind. Eye problems have spiritual as well as physiological causes. One aid, therefore, is *meiso*, or meditation, whereby all five senses are heightened, thus improving vision. Relaxation by means of self-suggestion and deep breathing is also effective.

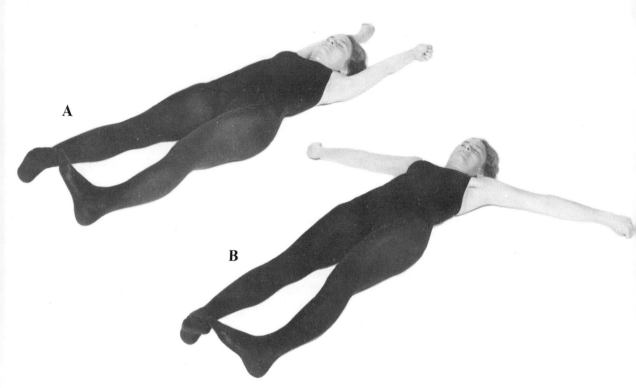

A

B

EXERCISE **30**

Myopia and Other Vison Problems 1

Starting Posture
Normal Breathing

Lie on the back, legs extended. Turn toes inward, pressing the big toes together, with heels apart.

Extend the arms overhead on the floor, palms up—spreading the arms shoulder width apart.

Relax in this posture briefly, then, inhale.

Extension
Exhaling

Twist the arms inward as much as possible so that the palms begin to face outward. Make fists. (Fig. A)

Pull the chin in. Stretch the Achilles tendons. Raise the feet about two to three inches off the floor.

Inhale deeply, then, retain the breath while holding this posture for a few seconds.

Corrective Movement
Exhaling

Close the eyes tightly. Tighten the fists. stretch the arms as much as possible. Move the feet up and down slowly, keeping the toes together and heels apart.

Raise the heels no higher than six to eight inches and do not let them drop to the floor.) Inhale, return to then starting posture and relax.

Repeat, varying the arm position at angles of 30 and 60 degrees below the original position as well as straight out to the side. (Fig. B)

EXERCISE **31**

Myopia and Other Vison Problems 2

Starting Posture
Normal Breathing

Lie on the back, bend the knees up and place the feet close to the buttocks. Keep the knees together and feet flat on the floor.

With the hands behind the head, place the thumbs directly behind the ear lobes at a point between the jaw bone and skull.

Relax in this posture briefly, then, inhale.

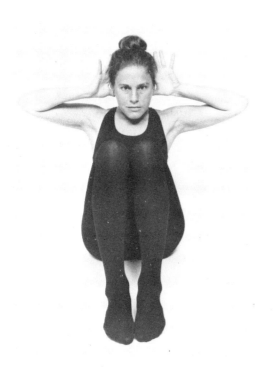

After you finish exhaling, hold this posture and retain the breath for a few seconds. Then, inhale, return to the starting posture and relax.

Repeat this exercise applying pressure with the thumbs to four different pairs of points:

FIRST, the points behind the ear lobes as described above.

SECOND, directly beneath the jaw on either side of the Adams apple (push upward)

THIRD, in the middle part of the throat directly beneath the second set of points.

FOURTH, along the side of the nostrils.

(Close the eyes tightly as you press on all of these points.

Extension

Exhaling

Keep the elbows on the floor, stretching them out to the sides. Pull the chin in and begin to apply pressure to the points.

Inhale deeply, then, retain the breath as you hold this posture for a few seconds.

Corrective Movement

Exhaling

Close the eyes tightly. Keeping the knees together, and pressing firmly behind the ears, sit up.

(Keep the elbows stretched, and the chin down.)

EXERCISE 32

Myopia and Other Vison Problems 3

Starting Posture

Normal Breathing

Sit up straight, legs extended and feet together. Turn the feet inward, pressing the big toes together, and spread the heels apart. Extend the arms forward at shoulder level. Interlock the fingers and turn the palms out. Relax in this posture briefly, then inhale.

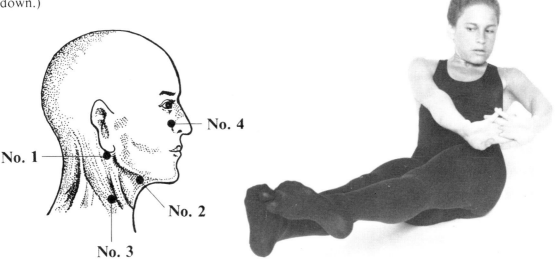

Extension
Exhaling

Pull the chin in. Stretch the Achilles tendons. Raise the feet six inches, while leaning the torso backwards.

(At this point, you should be balancing on the base of the spine. Take care not to bend the knees or the elbows).

Inhale deeply, then, retain the breath while holding this posture for a few seconds.

Corrective Movement
Exhaling

Slowly swing the legs to one side, turning the arms and the upper torso to the opposite side.

Continue, reversing directions.

(Keep the eyes focused on the toes, without turning the head in the direction of the feet.)

Inhale, return to the starting posture and relax.

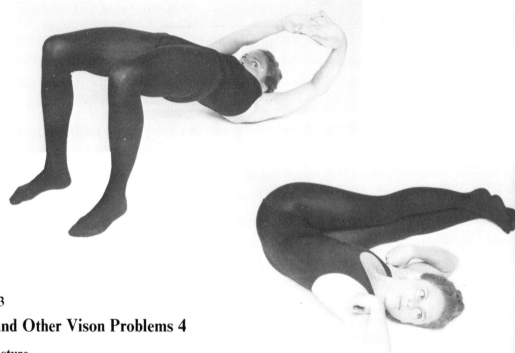

EXERCISE 33

Myopia and Other Vison Problems 4

Starting Posture
Normal Breathing

Lie on the back, legs extended and feet spread waist-width.

Extend the arms straight up, pointing to the ceiling. Interlock the fingers and turn the palms out.

Relax in this posture briefly, then, inhale.

Extension
Exhaling

Pulling the chin in, arch the chest and lift the hips. Stretch the arms up.

Alternate Posture

To make this exercise more effective; lift the shoulders off the floor and balance on the crown of the head; and press the knees together.

Inhale deeply, then, retain the breath while holding this posture for a few seconds.

Corrective Movement
Exhaling

Raise the hips up even further, slowly moving the arms as far as possible to one side, then, to the other.

Keep the hands at eye level. Move the eyes with the arms without turning the head.

(Keep the legs and hips stationary.)

Inhale, return to the starting posture and relax.

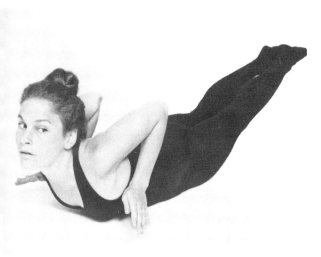

Myopia and Other Vison Problems 5

Starting Posture

Normal Breathing

Lie on the back, legs extended and feet together.

Make fists and place them under the arm pits, resting the elbows on the floor.

Relax in this posture briefly, then, inhale.

Extension

Exhaling

Keep the elbows on the floor, stretching them downward and out to the sides.

Pull the chin in. Stretch the Achilles tendons.

Raise the legs towards the ceiling.

Inhale deeply, then retain the breath while holding this posture for a few seconds.

Corrective Movement

Exhaling

Press the elbows down on the floor.

Slowly bring the legs to one side, stopping just short of the floor, without bending the knees.

At the same time, slowly turn the head to the opposite side.

Inhale, return to the starting position, and then turn the head and legs down to the opposite sides, as you exhale.

Inhale, return to the starting posture and relax.

Myopia and Other Vison Problems 6

Starting Posture

Normal Breathing

Lie on the stomach, legs extended, feet together and forehead on the floor.

Place the palms down, fingers pointing toward the head just below the shoulders.

Relax in this posture briefly, then, inhale.

Extension

Exhaling

Raise the hands and legs off the floor, arching the back as far as possible.

At the same time, squeeze the elbows together. Point your toes, relaxing the Achilles tendons.

Inhale deeply, then, retain the breath while holding this posture for a few seconds.

Corrective Movement

Exhaling

Swing the whole upper body from side to side as far as possible, while keeping the legs and hips stationary.

Move the eyes side to side with the body.

Inhale, return to the starting posture and relax.

Variation on Cobra Pose (*Practical Yoga*, p. 28).

Myopia and Other Vison Problems 7

Starting Posture

Normal Breathing

Lie on the stomach, legs extended, forehead on the floor. Spread the feet waist-width.

Extend the arms behind the back, clasping the hands, turning the palms out.

Relax in this posture briefly, then, inhale.

Extension

Exhaling

Stretch the arms up toward the head. With the Achilles tendons relaxed, raise the legs,

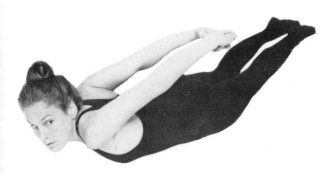

head and chest off the floor as high as possible.

Keep the knees straight.

Inhale deeply, then, retain the breath while holding this posture for a few seconds.

Corrective Movement

Exhaling

Slowly move the arms from side to side as far as possible.

At the same time, move the eyes in the same direction as the arms.

(Avoid turning the head as much as possible, while moving the eyes from side to side.)

Inhale, return to the starting posture and relax.

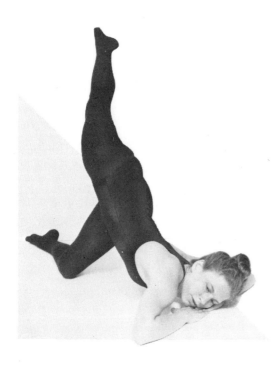

EXERCISE **37**

Myopia and Other Vison Problems 8

Starting Posture

Normal Breathing

Kneel on all fours with knees and feet together.

Place the hands on the floor, palms down, one on top of the other. Rest the chin on the hands.

Place the chest as close to the floor as possible.

Relax in this posture briefly, then, inhale.

Extension

Exhaling

Keep the elbows firmly on the floor, stretching them in out to the sides.

Raise one leg straight up as high as possible. Keep the knee straight and point the toes.

Inhale deeply, then retain the breath while holding this posture for a few seconds.

Corrective Movement

Exhaling

Press down on the floor with the elbows.

Slowly swing the extended leg as far as possible from side to side.

As you swing the extended leg:

1.) Press down with the opposite knee keeping the thigh perpendicular to the floor.

2.) Turn the head in the direction opposite to the swing of the leg, keeping the chin on the hands.

Inhale, return to the starting posture and relax.

Repeat the exercise with the opposite leg extended. Do the exercise more in the posture more difficult.

Variation on Twist Corrective Exercise No. 4 (*Practical Yoga*, p. 64).

Hardness of Hearing

Hardness of hearing is usually attributed to the aging process causing a degenerative condition in the external, middle or inner ear. However, the aged are not the only victims of hardness of hearing. Incorrect posture, affecting the nervous system, can cause tinnitus (ringing in the ears) or hardness of hearing in both young and old; in such cases, the auditory nerves become fatigued or disordered.

Likewise, the auditory nerves are sensitive to damage by various commonly used drugs. For example, streptomycin can lead to malfunction of the adrenal glands, which, in turn, can do damage to the autonomic nerves. Improper diet, which can harden the muscles and tissue of the auditory system, is another detriment to hearing ability.

Therefore, in order to heal ear problems, attention must be paid to diet, and drugs must not be used indiscriminately. Concurrently, exercise to correct posture and regulate the nervous system should be performed.

EXERCISE **38** **Hearing 1**

Starting Posture

Normal Breathing

Sit up with the back straight, legs extended, and feet together.

Place the left foot at the outside of the right knee; planting the sole of the foot firmly on the floor. Inhale.

Exhaling, turn the torso to the left.

Reach down and grasp the left calf with the right hand. Inhale. (At this point the right elbow is pressing against the outside of the left knee.)

Exhaling, bring the left hand around behind you so that the back of the hand is against the small of the back on the right hand side. Turn the head and torso as far as possible to the left.

Relax in this posture briefly, then, inhale.

Extension

Exhaling

Slowly turn your head and torso as far as possible to the left. (At this point, the back should still be vertical.)

Inhale deeply, then, retain the breath, while holding this posture for a few seconds.

Corrective Movement

Exhaling

Turn to the left even further and lean back toward the floor as far as possible.

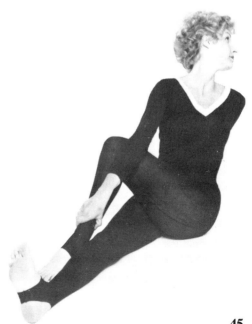

45

After you finish exhaling, hold this posture and retain the breath for a few seconds. Then, inhale, return to the starting posture and relax.

Repeat the exercise reversing the position of the arms and legs. Do more in the posture more difficult.

Variation on Twist Pose (*Practical Yoga*, p. 38)

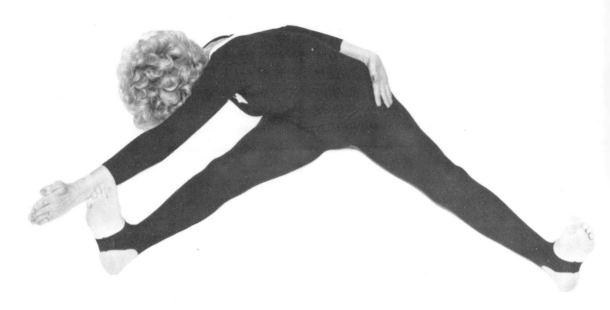

EXERCISE 39 Hearing 2

Starting Posture

Normal Breathing

Sit on the floor, legs extended, and feet spread apart as widely as possible.

Raise one arm directly overhead, palm facing inward.

Bring the other arm around behind you, placing the hand firmly on the opposite hip.

Relax in this posture briefly, then, inhale.

Extension

Exhaling

Pull the chin in. Stretch the Achilles tendons. Stretch the extended arm as much as possible while straightening the back.

Inhale deeply, then, retain the breath while holding this posture for a few seconds.

Corrective Movement

Exhaling

Bend the torso forward to the right side, trying to touch hand to foot and chest to knee.

Inhale, return to the starting position.

Bend forward in the same manner to the left side, as you exhale.

(As you bend forward, keep the raised arm pressed firmly against the ear and keep the opposite arm on the hip.)

Inhale, return to the starting posutre and relax.

Pepeat the excercise reversing the arms. Do more in the posture more difficult.

EXERCISE 40 Hearing 3

Starting Posture

Normal Breathing

Lie on the back, bringing the heels close to the buttocks, spread waist-width apart.

Bend the elbows to make the arms "L" shaped, fingertips in the direction of the feet.

Relax in this posture briefly, then, inhale.

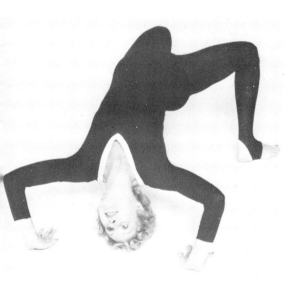

Extension

Exhaling

Raise the body up so that it is supported on the hands, feet and top of the head.

Inhale deeply, then retain the breath while holding this posture for a few seconds.

Corrective Movement

Exhaling

Arch the chest and hips upwards as high as possible.

Bend the head slowly from side to side so that the ears touch the shoulders.

Inhale, return to the starting posture and relax.

Variation on Arch Pose (*Practical Yoga*, p. 32)

EXERCISE **41 Hearing 4**

Starting Posture

Normal Breathing

Kneel on all fours, knees and feet together. Extend both arms straight out on the floor (palms down), hands spread apart slightly more than shoulder-width.

Place the chest on the floor.

Relax in this posture briefly, then, inhale.

Extension

Exhaling

Make fists and stretch the arms forward.

Without bending the knee, raise one leg off the floor as high as possible and relax the Achilles tendon.

Inhale deeply, then, retain the breath while holding this posture for a few seconds.

Corrective Movement

Exhaling

Pressing down on the floor with the arms, slowly swing the extended leg as far as possible from side to side.

At the same time, turn the head to the opposite side.

Press the opposite knee down firmly to avoid letting the hips fall from side to side while moving the extended leg.

Inhale, return to the starting posture and relax.

Repeat the exercise, reversing the positions of the legs, and do the exercise more in the posture more difficult for you.

Variation on Twist Corrective Exercise No. 4 (*Practical Yoga*, p. 65)

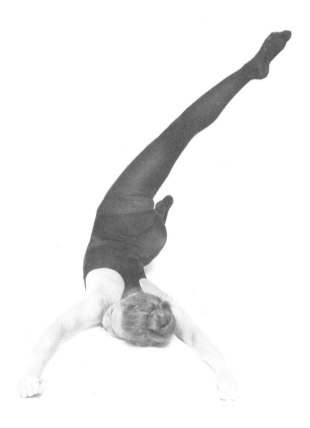

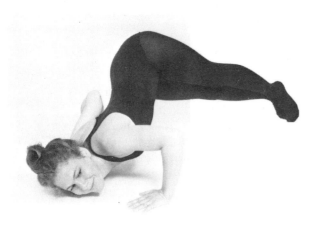

EXERCISE 42   Hearing 5

Starting Posture

Normal Breathing

Kneel on all fours, knees and feet together; and hands spread shoulder-width apart.
Relax in this posture briefly, then, inhale.

Extension

Exhaling

Raise the right leg and right arm. Extend them, holding them at a height even with the back.
Pull the chin in and relax the Achilles tendon. (Keep the right arm pressed tightly against the ear throughout the exercise.)
Inhale deeply, then, retain the breath while holding this posture for a few seconds.

Corrective Movement

Exhaling

Swing the right leg slowly to the left as far as possible. (Press the left knee firmly into the floor to keep the hips from falling to the side as you move the extended leg.)
After you finish exhaling, hold this posture and retain the breath for a few seconds. Then, inhale, return to the starting posture and relax.
Repeat the exercise reversing the positions of the legs, and do the exercise more in the posture more difficult for you.

EXERCISE 43   Hearing 6

Starting Posture

Normal Breathing

Lie on the stomach, legs extended, feet together, forehead on the floor.
Place the hands on the floor six inches off the side of the shoulders. Without moving the hands bring the elbows up to the level of the shoulders.
Relax in this posture briefly, then, inhale.

Extension

Exhaling

Raise the hips as high as possible, legs together, face and chest close to the floor.
Keeping the face and chest close to the floor, and the legs straight, raise the hips upward as high as possible.
Inhale deeply, then, retain the breath while holding this posture for a few seconds.

Corrective Movement

Exhaling

Slowly lower the hips from side to side, stopping just short of the floor.
Inhale, return to the starting posture and relax.
Variation on Distortion Corrective Exercise (*Practical Yoga*, p. 56)

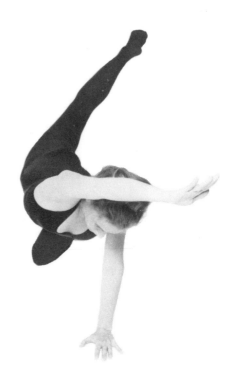

Fallen Stomach

Fallen stomach is a malfunctional stomach which droops down from its proper anatomical position. The life style which weakens the stomach, of course, contributes to falling of all the internal organs, therefore inviting dis-ease. Some symptoms of fallen stomach are abdominal ache, indigestion, belching, minor sore throat, loss of appetite, general fatigue, stiff shoulders and headache.

It has been observed that the fallen stomach type has rounded shoulders and back; the arms are weak, the foot muscles chronically contracted and the body weight falls full on the heels. Above all, there is little strength in tanden.

EXERCISE **44** **Fallen Stomach 1**

Starting Posture
Normal Breathing
Lie on the back, legs extended, feet together.
Extend the arms directly overhead. Clasp the hands, turning the palms outward.
Relax in this posture briefly, then, inhale.
Extension
Exhaling
Pull the chin in.
Press the knees together. Lift the hips up.

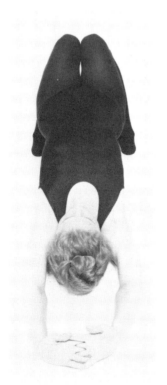

Stretch the Achilles tendons.
Inhale deeply, then, retain the breath while holding this posture for a few seconds.
Corrective Movement
Exhaling
Stretch the arms overhead in the direction of the head.
Move the hips up and down without touching the floor.
Inhale, return to the starting posture and relax.

EXERCISE **45** **Fallen Stomach 2**

Starting Posture
Normal Breathing
Lie on the back, legs extended and feet together. Inhale.
Exhaling, slowly raise the legs to the ceiling. Support the hips with both hands, inhaling.
Exhaling, bring the legs over the head parallel to the floor. Inhale.
Exhaling, bend the knees to forehead pointing the toes to the ceiling.
Relax in this posture briefly, then, inhale.
Extension
Exhaling
Pull the chin in. Stretch the Achilles tendons.

49

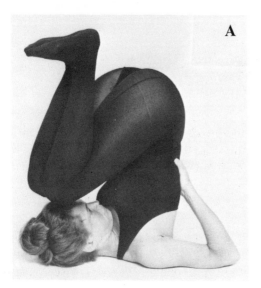

A   B

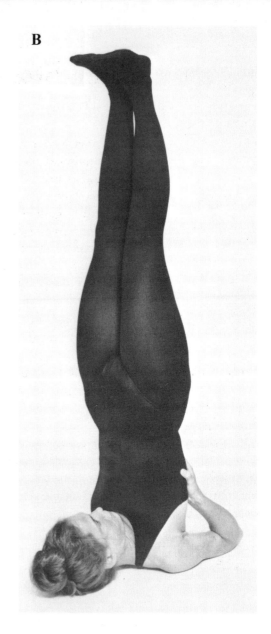

Place the elbows out to the sides.

Inhale deeply, then, retain the breath while holding this posture for a few seconds.

Corrective Movement

Exhaling

Stretch the legs straight up (Fig. B) and lower to the starting position (Fig. A).

Slowly move the legs up and down.

Inhale, return to the starting posture and relax.

Shoulder Stand Pose (*Prectical Yoga*, p. 20).

EXERSICE **46**   **Fallen Stomach 3**

Starting Posture

Normal Breathing

Lie on the stomach, legs extended, forehead on the floor, feet spread waist-width.

Join the palms together behind the back in prayer fashion (Gasho). Point the fingers toward the head.

Relax in this posture briefly, then, inhale.

Extension

Exhaling

Relax the Achilles tendons, raise the legs up as high as possible without bending the knees.

At the same time, move the hands as far as possible up the spine while arching the chest back.

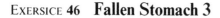

Inhale deeply, then, retain the breath while holding this posture for a few seconds.

Corrective Movement

Exhaling

Without bending the knees, move the legs up and down in unison, not letting the feet touch the floor.

50

Inhale, return to the starting posture and relax.

Variation on Cobra Pose (*Practical Yoga*, p. 28)

EXERCISE 47 **Fallen Stomach 4**

Starting Posture

Normal Breathing

Stand with legs spread one and a half times waist-width, feet parallel to each other.

Bend forward, keeping the knees straight. Place the hands on the floor, fingers spread apart, pointing forward.

(The arms should be straight and stretched out as far as possible in front of the shoulders).

Relax in this posture briefly, then, inhale.

Extension

Exhaling

Tuck the head back between the arms pushing the chin down against the chest.

Raise the hips up as high as possible (Fig. A).

Inhale deeply, then retain the breath while holding this posture for a few seconds.

Corrective Movement

Exhaling

With one motion, lower the hips near to the floor arching the head and upper torso up and back, keeping the arms straight. (Fig. B).

(At this point the face should be parallel to the ceiling and legs, and lower abdomen be only about two or three inches off the floor).

Inhale, returning to the starting posture and repeat, exhaling. Try to gradually increase the speed of movement.

Purification Exercise (*Practical Yoga* p. 73).

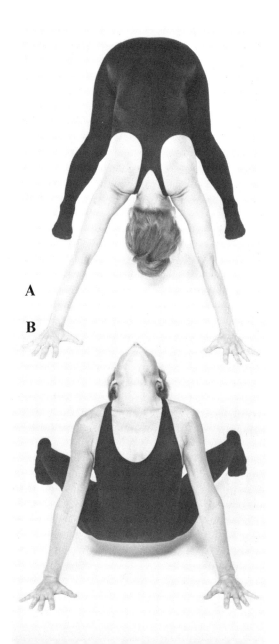

A

B

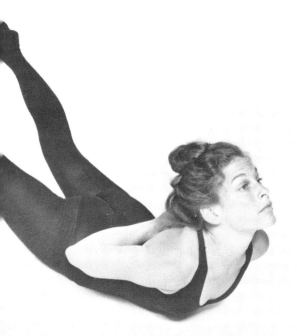

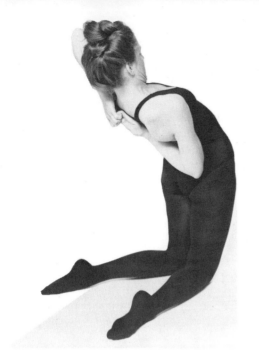

EXERCISE **48** **Fallen Stomach 5**

Starting Posture

Normal Breathing

Kneel with the knees together and feet spread waist-width.

Clasp the hands behind the back, bringing the left arm over the left shoulder, and the right arm from below.

Relax in this posture briefly then inhale.

Extension

Exhaling

Pull the chin in, press the knees together, and start to pull the fingers apart. (If clasping is not possible, use a towel.)

Inhale deeply, then, retain the breath as you hold this posture for a few seconds.

Corrective Movement

Exhaling

Keep the chin down.

Arch the back as far as possible, pushing the abdomen for ward. Pull strongly on the fingers.

Bend the upper torso from side to side.

After you finish exhaling, hold this posture and retain the breath for a few seconds. Then, inhale, return to the starting posture and relax.

Repeat the exercise reversing the position of the arms. Do exercise more in the posture more difficult.

EXERCISE **49** **Fallen Stomach 6**

Starting Posture

Normal Breathing

Lie on the stomach, legs extended, and feet together forehead on the floor.

Place the hands on the floor six inches to the sides of the shoulders, fingertips forward. Relax in this posture briefly, then, inhale.

Extension

Exhaling

Bring the elbows in close to the torso and raise one leg about one foot off the floor without bending the knee.

Inhale deeply, then, retain the breath while holding this posture for a few seconds.

Corrective Movement

Exhaling

Keeping the back of the neck extended and the raised leg stationary, push up slowly.

(Raise the chest only about six to eight inches off the floor and take care not to let the body touch the floor on the down motion.)

Inhale, return to the starting posture and relax.

Repeat the exercise raising the opposite leg. Do the exercise more in the posture more difficult.

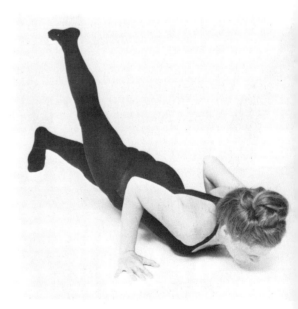

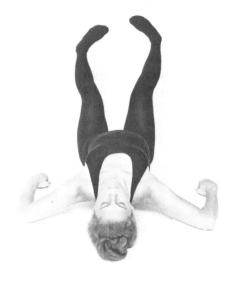

EXERCISE 50 Fallen Stomach 7

Starting Posture
Normal Breathing

Lie on the back, legs extended, and feet spread waist-width. Turn the toes inward. Bend the elbows down 'L' shaped on the floor fingers pointing down. Make fists.
Keep the upper arms shoulder height.
Relax in this posture briefly, then, inhale.

Extension
Exhaling

Keeping the arms on the floor, pull the elbows up towards the head.
Pull the chin in. Stretch the Achilles tendons. Raise the heels about three or four inches off the floor.
Inhale deeply, then, retain the breath while holding this posture for a few seconds.

Corrective Movement
Exhaling

Arching the lower back, slowly move the abdomen up and down. Continuing to pull the arms up, holding the legs in place.
As you repeat this arching movement, take care to:
1.) keep the lower back and legs raised.
2.) press down firmly with the arms as you raise the abdomen.
Inhale, return to the starting posture and relax.
Variation on Center of Gravity Exercise No. 3 (*Practical Yoga*, p. 67)

EXERCISE 51 Fallen Stomach 8

Starting Posture
Normal Breathing

Lie on the back, right leg extended and left leg bent back at the knee, left foot next to the hip.
Place the right hand in the stomach.
Grasp the left ankle with the left hand.
Relax in this posture briefly, then, inhale.

Extension
Exhaling

Pull the chin in; stretch the Achilles tendon of the extended leg; pull up on the ankle.
Inhale deeply, then, retain the breath while holding this posture for a few seconds.

Corrective Movement
Exhaling

Sit-up to a position 90 degrees from the floor. At the same time, apply pressure to the stomach, pushing down with the right hand. After you finish exhaling, hold this posture and retain the breath for a few seconds. Then, inhale, return to the starting posture and relax.
Repeat the exercise with the left leg extended and do the exercise more in the posture more difficult.
Variation on Pelvis Strengthening Exercise No. 4 (*Practical Yoga*, p. 55)

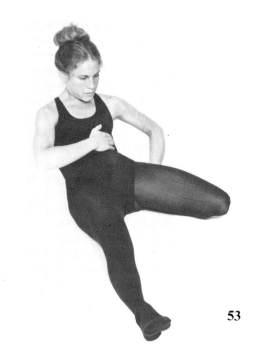

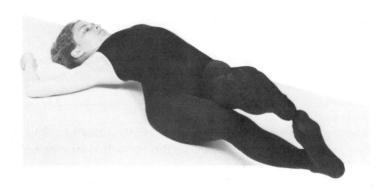

EXERCISE 52   Fallen Stomach 9

Starting Posture
Normal Breathing

Lie on the back, legs extended, left heel on the right toes.

Without moving the hips, move the legs several inches to the right.

Keeping the arms on the floor, bend the elbows 'L' shaped, fingers pointing in the direction of the head. Make loose fists.

Relax in this posture briefly, then, inhale.

Extension
Exhaling

Arch the lower back, pressing the arms firmly on the floor. Stretch the Achilles tendons.

Inhale deeply, then, retain the breath while holding this posture for a few seconds.

Corrective Movement
Exhaling

Slowly move the legs up and down, without bending the knees.

(As you do this the heels should raise only three to four inches off the floor. Do not touch the floor with the feet.)

Inhale, return to the starting posture and relax.

EXERCISE 53   Fallen Stomach 10

Starting Posture
Normal Breathing

Lie on the stomach, legs extended, feet together.

Join the hands together behind the back in prayer fashion, fingers pointing to the head. Bend the right knee, bringing the right foot close to the left thigh.

Relax in this posture briefly, then, inhale.

Extension
Exhaling

Move the hands further up the spine, while moving the right knee up toward the head. Stretch the Achilles tendon in the left leg.

Inhale deeply, then, retain the breath while holding this posture for a few seconds.

Corrective Movement
Exhaling

Arch the chest, bringing the face parallel to the ceiling.

Raise the left leg as high as possible without bending the knee. (Continue to move the hands up the spine as you raise the torso and leg.)

After you finish exhaling, hold this posture and retain the breath for a few seconds. Then, inhale, return to the starting posture and relax.

Repeat the exercise reversing the position of the legs. Do the exercise more in the posture more difficult.

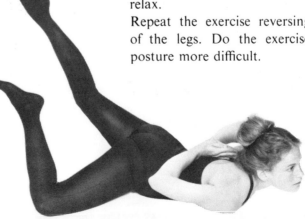

Sinus and Nasal Problems

Most nasal problems are caused by postural distortion, misalignment and improper diet. Common to all nasal and sinus problems are a condition in which the nasal membrane is inflamed and infected, and, oftentimes, the olfactory sense numbed. Headache, stuffy nose and nasal mucus of an unpleasant odor result.

It has been observed that those with nasal problems bear the body weight too much on the heels and outsides of the feet; the ankles tend to be weak. Asana such as the arch, cobra and fish poses (described in *Practical Yoga*) are very effective. Shusei taiso which intends to extend the shorter leg, properly align the cervicals and strengthen the ankles is recommended.

To reap further benefit, massage the sides of the nose upwards from the base to the bridge while doing the exercise. Nasal douching with saltwater or vegetable juice is also helpful.

EXERCISE **54** **Sinus 1**

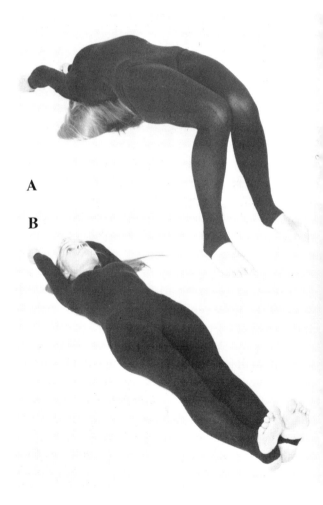

A

B

Starting Posture

Normal Breathing

Lie on the back, legs extended, and feet spread six inches apart.

Extend the arms directly overhead, palms facing inward, biceps pressing against the ears.

Relax in this posture briefly, then, inhale.

Extension

Exhaling

Pull the chin in. Make fists.

Support on the top of the head, raising the torso and hips off the floor. (At this point only the head, hands and feet are touching the floor).

Inhale deeply, then retain the breath while holding this posture for a few seconds.

Corrective Movement

Exhaling

1) Press the knees together, stretch the arms up even further, and arch the body up as high as possible as you exhale (Fig. A).
2) Let the entire body drop to the floor suddenly (Fig. B).

Inhale and relax in the starting posture.

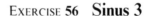

EXERCISE 55　Sinus 2

Starting Posture
Normal Breathing
Kneel with the knees together and the feet spread to waist-width.
Reach back and grasp the outside of the ankles, leaning back slowly. Resting the back of the head on the floor.
Relax in this posture briefly, then, inhale.
Extension
Exhaling
Begin to pull up on the ankles as you arch up on to the top of the head.
(Keep the knees together and the arms straight.)
Inhale deeply, then, retain the breath while holding this posture for a few seconds.
Corrective Movement
Exhaling
Slowly turn the head from side to side, stretching the neck as far as possible.
Inhale, return to the starting posture and relax.
Variation on Arch Pose (*Practical Yoga*, p. 32)

EXERCISE 56　Sinus 3

Starting Posture
Normal Breathing
Lie on the back, legs extended and feet together.
Arms at sides, bend at the elbows so that your hands pointing to the ceiling. Make fists.
Relax in this posture briefly, then, inhale.
Extension
Exhaling
Stretch the Achilles tendons. Arch the back off the floor; supporting on the top of the head and elbows.
Inhale deeply, then, retain the breath while holding this posture for a few seconds.
Corrective Movement
Exhaling
Press down on the floor with the elbows. Slowly turn the feet and the head from side to side.
First perform this movement, turning the head and feet in the same direction. Then repeat the exercise turning the head and feet in opposite directions.
Inhale, return to the starting posture and relax.
Basic Fish Pose (*Practical Yoga*, p. 22)

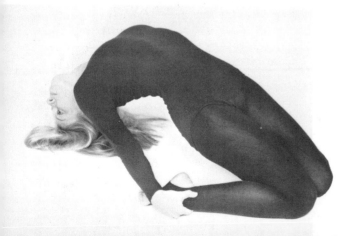

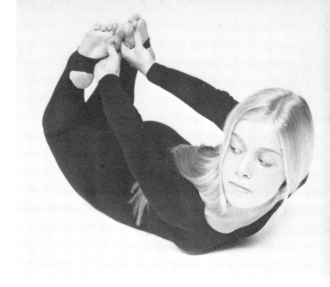

EXERCISE 57   Sinus 4

Starting Posture
Normal Breathing

Lie on the stomach, legs extended, feet together, forehead on the floor.

Bending the knees, bring the feet up toward the head. Reach back and grasp the ankles from the inside.

Relax in this posture briefly, then, inhale.

Extension
Exhaling

Press the knees together tightly. Pull the feet towards the head, raising the head and upper body off the floor as high as possible. Lift the chin up.

Inhale deeply, then, retain the breath while holding this posture for a few seconds.

Corrective Movement
Exhaling

Maintaining this posture, slowly turn the head from side to side. Stretch as far as possible in both directions.

Inhale, return to the starting posture and relax.

Variation on Bow Pose (*Practical Yoga*, p. 26)

EXERCISE 58   Sinus 5

Starting Posture
Normal Breathing

Lie on the back, the soles of the feet together and slide the heels up close to the buttocks.

Place the fingertips on the sides of the nose —at about the middle of the nose. (Do not squeeze the nostrils.)

Relax in this posture briefly, then, inhale.

Extension
Exhaling

Push the elbows, keeping them on the floor. Pressing the knees down to the floor. Pull the chin in.

Apply pressure to the sides of the nose, pushing upwards towards the bridge of the nose.

Inhale deeply, then, retain the breath while holding this posture for a few seconds.

Corrective Movement
Exhaling

Sit-up, as you pressing firmly on the sides of the nose. (Continue to stretch the elbows out to the sides keeping the chin pulled in.) After you finish exhaling, hold this posture and retain the breath for a few seconds. Then, inhale, return to the starting posture and relax.

Variation on Pelvic Strengthening Exercise No. 4 (*Practical Yoga*, p. 55)

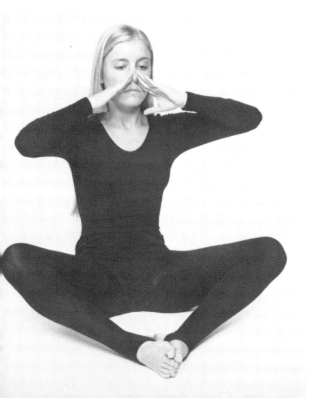

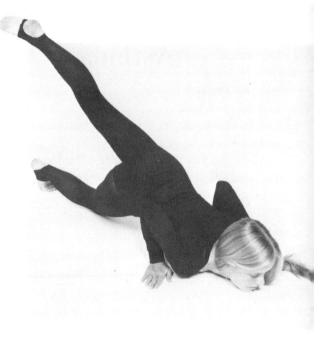

EXERCISE 59   Sinus 6

Starting Posture

Normal Breathing

Kneel on all fours with knees and feet together, hands on the floor, and shoulder width apart.

Lower the chin and chest to the floor.

Relax in this posture briefly, then, inhale.

Extension

Exhaling

Bring the elbows in close to the body and raise one leg straight up without bending the knee.

Inhale deeply, then, retain the breath while holding this posture for a few seconds.

Corrective Movement

Exhaling

Without moving the head and arms, slowly swing the extended leg from side to side, stopping just short of the floor.

Inhale, return to the starting posture and relax.

Repeat the exercise raising and moving the opposite leg. Do the exercise more in the posture more difficult.

EXERCISE 60   Sinus 7

Starting Posture

Normal Breathing

Kneel, knees together, feet spread apart one and a half times waist-width.

Place the hands on the sides of the face with the heels of the hands under the chin.

Keep the elbows spread apart.

Relax in this posture briefly, then, inhale.

Extension

Exhaling

Lean back, pushing up on the chin. (At this point, the elbows should be pointing up toward the ceiling.)

Inhale deeply, then, retain the breath while holding this posture for a few seconds.

Corrective Movement

Exhaling

Pushing the chin and head back as far as possible, arch the chest and push the hips forward. (This exercise is more effective if you open the mouth widely and exhaling forcefully.)

After you finish exhaling, hold this posture and retain the breath for a few seconds. Then, inhale, return to the starting posture and relax.

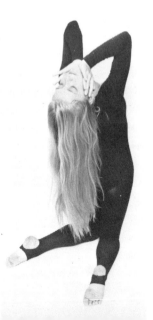

Asthma

The coughing that accompanies asthma is only a symptom of dis-ease. Coughing is, in fact, a healing process to eliminate mucus from the bronchiales, promoting clear air flow. Duriful taking of drugs to relieve spasm can have adverse effects and should be avoided. If coughing persists, however, a physical examination is advised, as the spasms could be caused by some other dis-ease such as bronchitis, pneumonia or lung cancer.

High emotion often initiates an attack, as the neck muscles harden during an emotionally excited state, causing tension and blockage. Gas-producing constipation, which irritates the throat, can also set off an attack.

The most common forms of asthma are bronchial and cardiac. Bronchial asthma often stems from allergy and malfunction of the autonomic nerves: the bronchiales are numbed, pleurae blood-congested, the air-sac is atrophied and mucus accumulates. Slow exhalation relieves discomfort. However, cardiac asthma is unaffected by such breathing. In cardiac asthma, the mucus is dry and attacks usually occur during sleep. While rest is absolutely imperative for cardiac asthma, vigorous exercise, fasting, cold-water bathing and zazen are measures to heal bronchial asthma.

The most common distortion found in asthma cases is that of the thoracic-cervical area, where congested blood accumulates. Breathing is inefficient, thus insufficiently exercising the lungs and not purging mucus. So, attacks result. Unfortunately, during a severe or prolonged attack (*status asthmeticus*) there is nothing to be done medically to assist.

When asthma registers at an early age, coughing attacks tend to disappear in time. If, however, the asthma persists, it most likely will become chronic, indicated by a protruding chest. Once that physical distortion is set, healing is less likely. Therefore, it is important to heal asthma early on.

EXERCISE 61   Asthma 1

Starting Posture

Normal Breathing

Lie on the stomach, legs extended, feet together, and forehead on the floor.

Extend the arms straight overhead, palms down. (The hands should be only a few inches apart.) Make fists.

Relax in this posture briefly, then, inhale.

Extension

Exhaling

Relaxing the Achilles tendons.

Stretch one arm out in front of the other, keeping both arms on the floor.

Inhale deeply, then, retain the breath while holding this posture for a few seconds.

Corrective Movement

Exhaling

Pressing down on the floor with the fists and the forehead, slowly raise both legs off the floor as high as possible without bending the knees.

Hold this posture and retain the breath for a few seconds. Then, inhale, return to the starting posture and relax.

Repeat the exercise stretching the opposite arm forward.

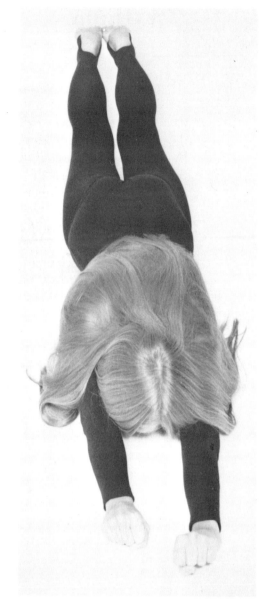

EXERCISE 62   Asthma 2

Strating posture and extension of this exercise are the same as in exercise 61.

Corrective Movement

Exhaling

Pressing down on the floor with the legs, continue to stretch the arms outward. Slowly raise the head, arms and chest off the floor as high as possible. (Lift the fact toward the ceiling).

Hold this posture and retain the breath for a few seconds. Then, inhale, return to the starting posture and relax.

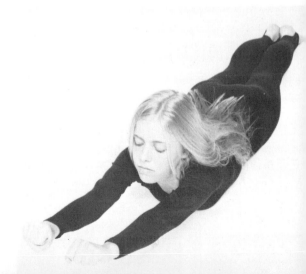

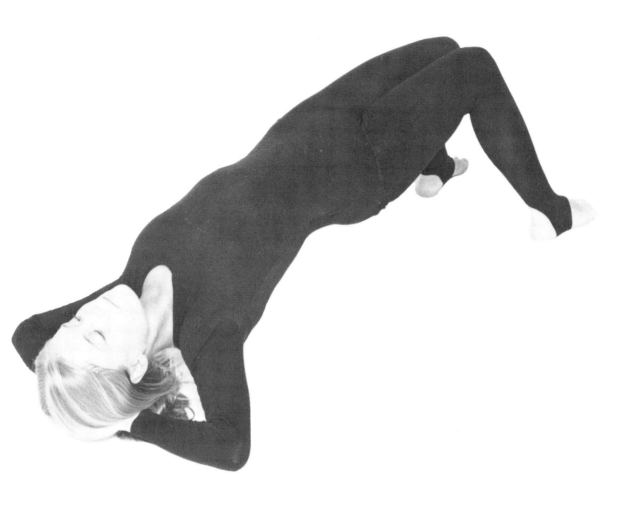

Exercise 63 Asthma 3

Starting Posture
Normal Breathing
Lie on the back, knees bent and feet spread waist-width apart.

Clasp your hands behind the head just above neck and rest the elbows on the floor.

Relax in this posture briefly, then, inhale.

Extension
Exhaling
Keeping the elbows on the floor, stretch them out to the sides.

Arch the chest up and raise hips off the floor. (At this point only the head, arms and the soles of the feet rest on the floor.)

Inhale deeply, then, retain the breath while holding this posture for a few seconds.

Corrective Movement
Exhaling
Remaining in this arched posture, alternately tense and relax the body in the following manner:

A.) Exhaling, pull the chin in, press the knees together and lift the body upward as high as possible.

B.) Inhale and slightly relax in the extension position.

Continue to tense and relax the body in this manner for as long as possible. Then inhale, return to the starting posture and relax.

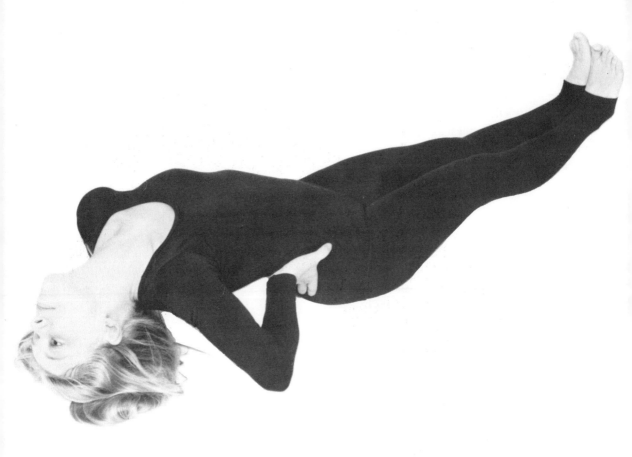

EXERCISE 64   Asthma 4

Starting Posture
Normal Breathing
Lie on the back, legs extended and feet together.
Slide the hands under the back just above the waist, resting the elbows on the floor.
Relax in this posture briefly, then, inhale.
Extension
Exhaling
Pull the chin in. Stretch the Achilles tendons. Support with the top of the head and the elbows, arching the back off the floor.
Inhale deeply, then, retain the breath while holding this posture for a few seconds.
Corrective Movement
Exhaling
Raise the legs three to four inches off the floor without bending the knees.
Prolong the exhalation and hold the legs up for as long as possible.

Hold this posture and retain the breath for a few seconds. Then, inhale, return to the starting posture and relax.

EXERCISE 65   Asthma 5

Starting Posture
Normal Breathing
Lie on the back. Bring the knees up close to the chest. Crasp the hands around the knees.
Relax in this posture briefly, then, inhale.
Extension
Exhaling
Pull the chin in. Stretch the Achilles tendons. Pull the knees together against the chest (Fig. A).
Inhale deeply, then retain the breath while holding this posture for a few seconds.

Corrective Movement

Exhaling

Try to straighten the legs and at the same time resist this effort by continuing to pull the knees against the chest (Fig. B).

(By resisting your own effort in this way, the head and neck will raise up off the floor slightly. But avoid doing a rocking motion. Instead, stretch the legs forward as you slowly exhale, keeping a balance between the opposing tensions in the arms and legs. When you do this movement properly, you will feel the tension centered in the chest.) Hold this posture and retain the breath for a few seconds. Then, inhale, return to the starting posture and relax.

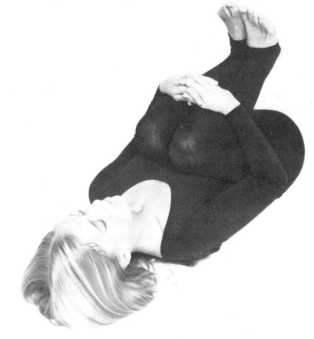

A

B

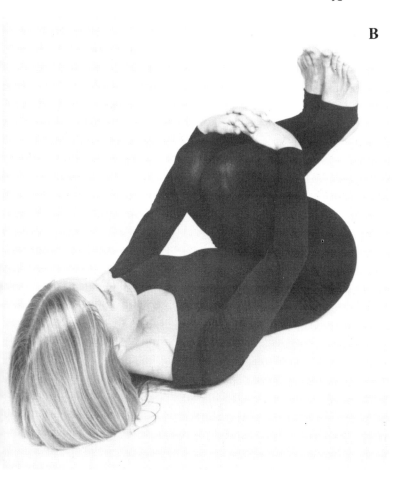

Exercise 66 Asthma 6

Starting Posture

Normal Breathing

Lie on the stomach with the feet resting on some object which is about a foot to a foot and a half high. Keep the legs straight and feet together (Fig. A).

Place the hands on the floor next to ribcage, about two inches below the shoulders.

Relax in this posture briefly, then, inhale.

Extension

Exhaling

Pull the chin in. Stretch the Achilles tendons. Inhale deeply, then, retain the breath while holding this posture for a few seconds.

Corrective Movement

Exhaling

Slowly push-up the body off the floor—until the arms are straight. Keep the back and legs straight and lift the face toward the ceiling.

Hold this posture and retain the breath

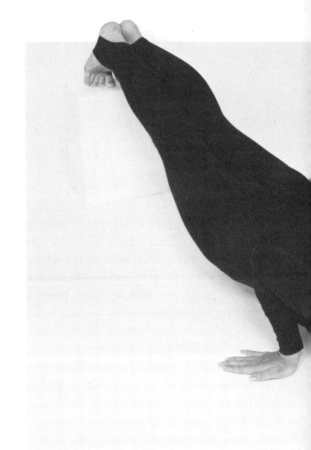

A

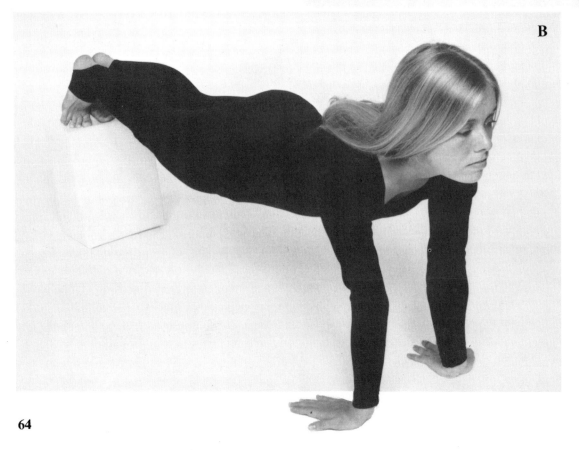

B

64

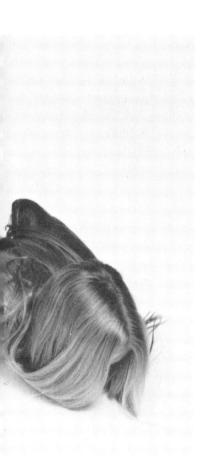

for a few seconds. Then, inhale, return to the starting posture and repeat the push-up motion several times.

Repeat the exercise with the hands in each of four different positions as follows:

Direction of the hands	Areas of stimulation
1. pointed to the feet	lower back
2. pointed to the head	neck
3. pointed inward	chest
4. pointed outward	upper back

EXERCISE 67 Asthma 7

Starting Posture
Normal Breathing
Kneel, spreading the knees to one and a half times waist-width.
Slowly lean back, without dropping the hips all the way to the floor.
Grasp the ankles, thumbs on the outside.
Relax in this posture briefly, then inhale.

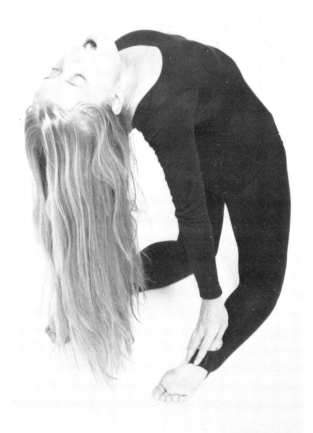

Extension
Exhaling

Straightening the arms, stretch the head back as far as possible.

At the same time, open the mouth as wide as possible and stick out the tongue.

Inhale deeply, then, retain the breath while holding this posture for a few seconds.

Corrective Movement
Exhaling

Slowly arch back the chest, extending the hips forward as far as possible.

Hold this posture and retain the breath for a few seconds. Then, inhale, return to the starting posture and relax.

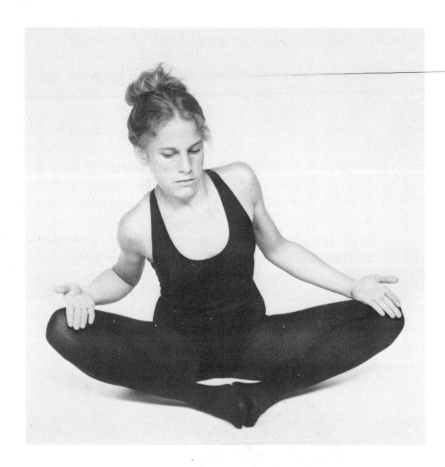

EXERCISE 68   Asthma 8

Starting Posture
Normal Breathing

Sitting on the floor, join the soles of the feet together and bring the heels close to buttocks. Grasp toes.

Relax in this posture briefly, then, inhale.

Extension
Exhaling

Pulling in the chin, straighten the back and arms. Spread the knees apart.

Inhale deeply, then retain the breath while holding this posture for a few seconds.

Corrective Movement
Exhaling

Bend forward slowly trying to touch the forehead to the floor. (Relax the shoulder.)

Hold this posture and retain the breath for a few seconds. Then, inhale, return to the starting posture and relax.

Bed-wetting

Some children continue past the normal age of control to urinate while sleeping. Causes of bed-wetting are both physiological and psychological; the latter are much more difficult to eliminate.

In daily situations, parents should reevaluate their relationship with children, and train them appropriately. Simply stated, bed-wetting generally persists so long as parents habitually awaken children during the night in order to urinate. Children must be taught a rhythmic and orderly way of life, deriving joy from living each moment while being aware that they may look forward to the future. There is, then, an appropriate time for every action. Such is the way of the religious mind cherished by Oki sensei.

EXERCISE **69** **Bed-wetting 1**

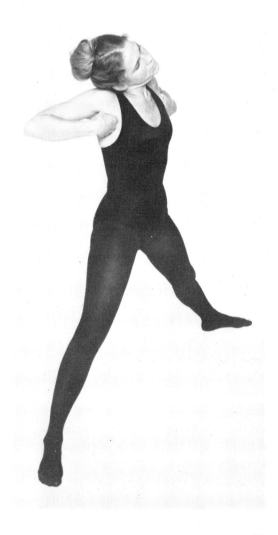

Starting Posture

Normal Breathing

Stand with the feet spread two or two and a half times the waist-width.

Make loose fists and place them under the armpits.

Keep the face forward and the back straight.

Relax in this posture briefly, then, inhale.

Extension

Exhaling

Pulling the chin in, stretch the elbows up and back, expanding the ribcage.

Inhale deeply, then, retain the breath while holding this posture for a few seconds.

Corrective Movement

Exhaling

Keeping the shoulders at the same level, bend the neck from side to side until the ear touches the shoulder.

Hold this posture and retain the breath for a few seconds. Then, inhale, return to the starting posture and relax.

This exercise will be more effective if you keep the feet parallel. This will help you to keep the back straight and will create more stimulation in the lower torso.

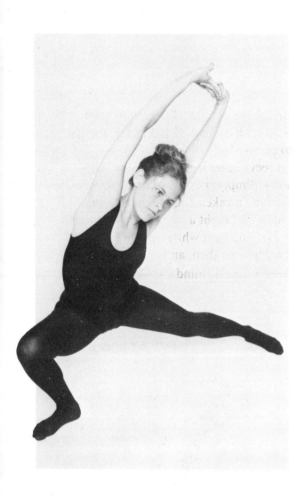

Corrective Movement

Exhaling

Continue to stretch the arms and upper body in the direction of the extended leg. Bend the opposite leg more, putting the weight in this leg.

After you finish exhaling, hold this posture and retain the breath for a few seconds. Then, inhale, return to the starting posture and relax.

Reverse the position of the legs and repeat the exercise, stretching to the opposite side. Do the exercise more in the posture more difficult for you.

EXERCISE 71 **Bed-wetting 3**

This exercise consists of three forward bending to the right foot, to the left foot, and to the center.

Starting Posture

Normal Breathing

Sit on the floor, legs spread apart as much as as possible.

Extend the arms to the ceiling. Interlock the fingers and turn the palms outward.

Relax in this posture briefly, then, inhale.

Extension

Exhaling

Pull the chin in. Stretch the Achilles tendons. Stretch the arms upward.

Inhale deeply, then, retain the breath while holding this posture for a few seconds.

Corrective Movement

Exhaling

Keeping your face and torso forward and the arms stretched upward. Bend forward to the right trying to touch your hands to the right foot.

Repeat, bending to the left and to the center. After each forward bend, hold this posture and retain the breath briefly before inhaling and returning to the starting posture.

EXERCISE 70 **Bed-wetting 2**

Starting Posture

Normal Breathing

Stand with the feet spread two to two and a half times waist-width.

Point one foot forward, keeping this leg straight, and point the other foot outwards, bending this leg outward.

Extend the arms up to the ceiling. Clasp the hands and turn the palms outward.

Relax in this posture briefly, then, inhale.

Extension

Exhaling

Pull the chin in. Bend in the direction of the extended leg, stretching the opposite side of the upper torso.

Inhale deeply, then, retain the breath while holding this posture for a few seconds.

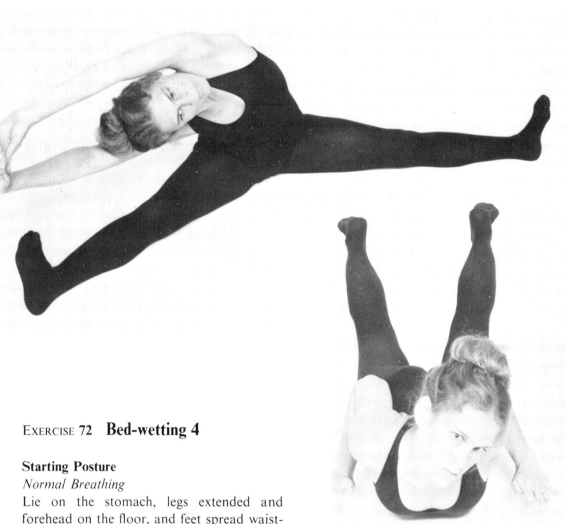

EXERCISE 72 Bed-wetting 4

Starting Posture
Normal Breathing
Lie on the stomach, legs extended and forehead on the floor, and feet spread waist-width apart.

Place the hands on the floor next to the ribcage, just below the shoulders.

Relax in this posture briefly, then, inhale.

Extension
Exhaling
Do the following movements simultaneously:
Upper Body;
Arch the chest off the floor as high as possible, trying to being the face parallel to the ceiling.
Keeping the hands parallel to the floor, lift the arms along with the head and chest.
Lower Body;
Raise the legs off the floor as high as possible without bending the knees.
Inhale deeply, then, retain breath while holding this posture for a few seconds.

Corrective Movement
Exhaling
Keep arms close to the body. Stretching one side of your ribcage, bend the upper body to the opposite direction.
Inhale, and then move the legs and upper body as you exhale—but this time in an up and down fashion.
Rock the upper body and legs alternately.
Inhale, return to the starting posture and relax.
Variation on Cobra Pose (*Practical Yoga*, p. 29)

EXERCISE 73 **Bed-wetting 5**

Starting Posture
Normal Breathing

Lie on the stomach, legs extended, forehead on the floor, and feet spread waist-width apart.

Bending the knees, bring the feet up toward the head. Reach back and grasp the ankles on the inside.

Relax in this posture briefly, then, inhale.

Extension
Exhaling

Lifting the face toward the ceiling, arch the chest back as far as possible.

Pull up on the ankles so that the knees come off the floor.

Inhale, return to the starting posture and relax.

Corrective Movement
Exhaling

Swing side to side.

Inhale, return to the starting posture and relax.

Variation on Bow Pose (*Practical Yoga*, p. 27)

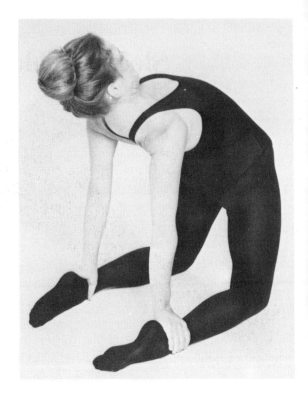

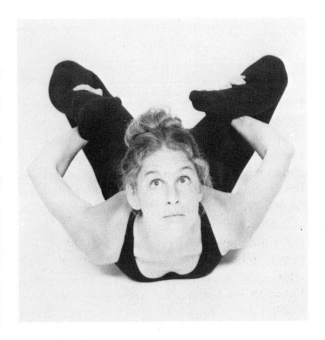

EXERCISE 74 **Bed-wetting 6**

Starting Posture
Normal Breathing

Kneel, feet spread to one and a half times waist-width.

Slowly lean back without dropping the hips to the floor. Grasp your ankles with the thumb on the inside.

Relax in this posture briefly, then, inhale.

Extension
Exhaling

Pull the chin in. Straightening the arms, stretch the head back as far as possible.

Inhale deeply, then, retain the breath while holding this posture for a few seconds.

Corrective Movement
Exhaling

Slowly arch the torso by expanding the chest, and extending the hips forward as far as possible.

After you finish exhaling, hold this posture and retain the breath for a few seconds. Then, inhale, return to the starting posture and relax.

Sleep Problems: Snoring and Grinding of the Teeth

When a person begins to snore without having previously done so, it is probable that some related dis-ease is brewing. People who snore have shifted their weight to the upper body; the shoulders and neck are tense; and both the cervicals and lumbars are rotationally misaligned.

Grinding of the teeth is common among people who suffer muscle spasm. Both are caused by an excessively alkaline condition.

By relaxing the neck muscles, balancing the bones of the skull, and aligning the rotational posture distortion, these sleep problems can be healed.

EXERCISE 75

Snoring and Grinding 1

Starting Posture
Normal Breathing

Lie on the back, joining the soles of the feet together. Bring the heels close to the buttocks. (The exercise can also be done with the legs crossed in the full lotus position.)
Bend the elbows 'L' shaped, fingers pointing to the ceiling. Make fists. Keep elbows close to the ribcage.
Relax in this posture briefly, then, inhale.

Extension
Exhaling

Pressing down on the floor with the elbows, arch the back off the floor and raise up on the top of the head.
Inhale deeply, then, retain the breath while holding this posture for a few seconds.

Corrective Movement
Exhaling

Press the right knee in to the floor. Turn the head slowly to the left; press the left knee down and turn the head slowly to the right. (Take care not to let the head drop to the floor and continue to arch the chest up as much as possible.)
Inhale, return to the starting posture and relax.

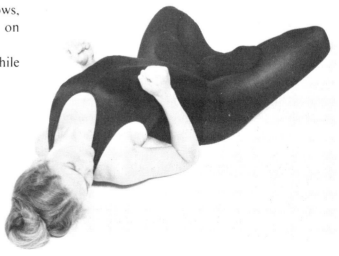

Snoring and Grinding 2

Starting Posture

Normal Breathing

Lie on the back, legs extended, and feet together.

Clasp your hands behind the neck and let the elbows rest on the floor.

Relax in this posture briefly, then, inhale.

Extension

Exhaling

Keeping the elbows down on the floor, stretch them out to the sides.

Squeeze the back of the head with the heels of the hands.

Pull the chin in. Stretch the Achilles tendons and raise the legs three or four inches off the floor.

Inhale deeply, then, retain the breath while holding this posture for a few seconds.

Corrective Movement

Exhaling

Move the legs up and down slowly without touching the floor.

At the same time, rotate the head slowly from side to side, stretching the back of the neck.

Inhale, return to the starting posture and relax.

Snoring and Grinding 3

Starting Posture

Normal Breathing

Lie on the back, legs extended and feet together.

Stretch the arms outward at shoulder level, palms down. Make fists.

Relax in this posture briefly, then, inhale.

Extension

Exhaling

Without bending the knees, raise the legs to the ceiling.

Pull the chin in. Stretch the Achilles tendons. Inhale deeply, the retain the breath while holding this posture for a few seconds.

Corrective Movement

Exhaling

Press down on the floor with the fists. Slowly

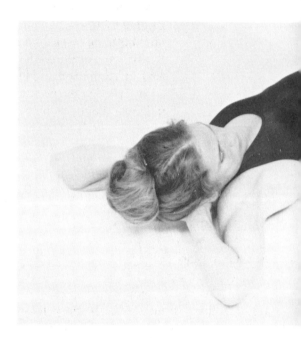

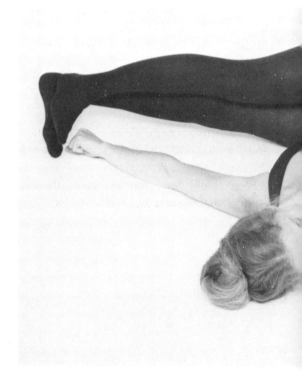

lower the legs to one side while turning the head slowly to the opposite side. Inhale, return to the starting posture and relax. Repeat to the opposite side.

EXERCISE **78**

Snoring and Grinding 4

Starting Posture
Normal Breathing
Lie on the stomach, legs extended, and feet together.
Place your hands on the floor close to the

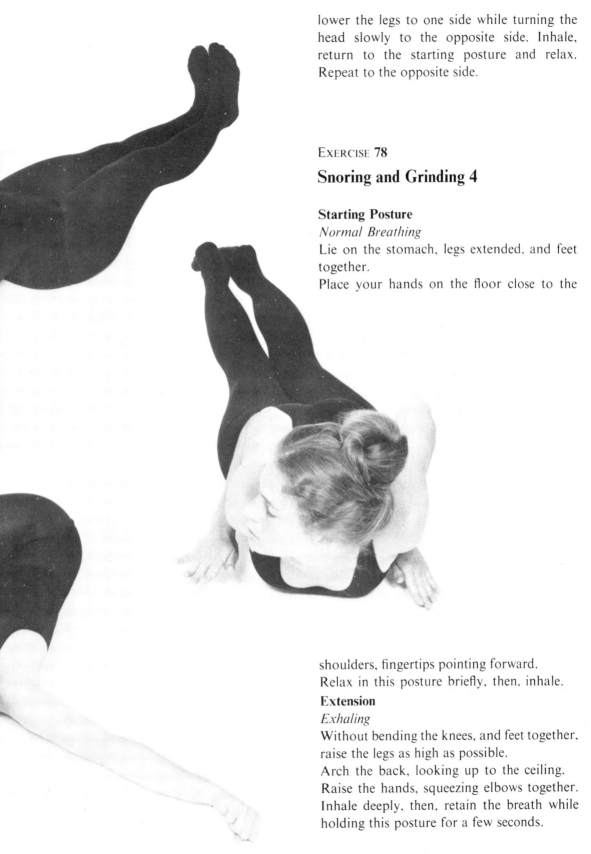

shoulders, fingertips pointing forward.
Relax in this posture briefly, then, inhale.
Extension
Exhaling
Without bending the knees, and feet together, raise the legs as high as possible.
Arch the back, looking up to the ceiling.
Raise the hands, squeezing elbows together.
Inhale deeply, then, retain the breath while holding this posture for a few seconds.

Corrective Movement

Exhaling

Slowly swing the legs as far as possible from one side to the other.

Move the legs in the same direction at the same time, trying to turn the head far enough to allow you to see the feet.

Inhale, return to the starting posture and relax.

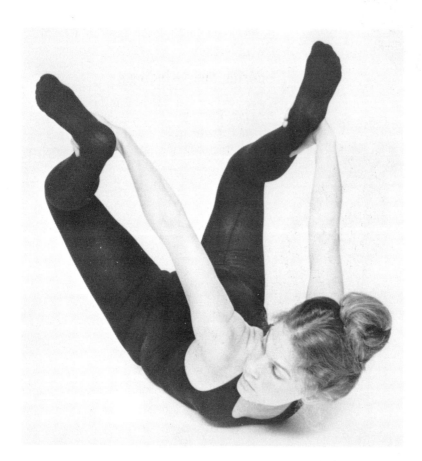

EXERCISE **79**

Snoring and Grinding 5

Starting posture and extension of this exercise are the same as in exercise 73.

Corrective Movement

Exhaling

Move the neck at random, noticing areas of stiffness.

Repeat with each of four "hand on ankle" position.

1. on the inside
2. on the outside
3. one hand on the inside; the other on the outside
4. reverse of 3.

To make the exercise most effective for you, determine which posture causes you the most difficulty and do the exercise in that posture.

Stuttering

For some people, when in an emotionally excited state, body weight shifts heavily to the upper body while the neck and shoulders tense; oftentimes, then, they stammer. Chronic cases of this physiological condition have been observed in stutterers, who, in addition, have twisted cervical vertebrae. As they try not to stutter, the neck and shoulders become even more tense, perpetuating dis-ease. By practicing tanden breathing and stretching the Achilles tendons, stutterers can achieve a proper body weight distribution and spinal alignment to relax the upper body.

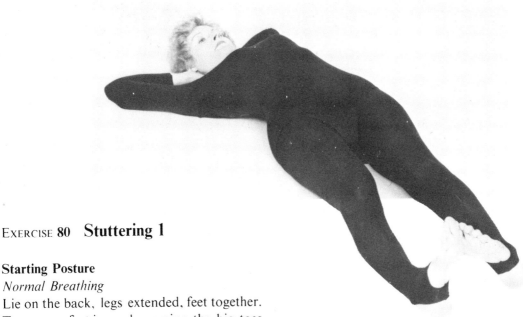

EXERCISE 80   Stuttering 1

Starting Posture
Normal Breathing
Lie on the back, legs extended, feet together. Turn your feet inward, pressing the big toes together, and heels spread.
Clasp the hands together behind the neck and rest the elbows on the floor.
Relax in this posture briefly, then, inhale.

Extension
Exhaling
Keep the elbows on the floor, stretched out to the sides. Raise the heels two or three inches.
Pull the chin in. Stretch the Achilles tendons. Inhale deeply, then, retain the breath while holding this posture for a few seconds.

Corrective Movement
Exhaling
Swing the legs slowly from side to side without bending the knees.
Inhale, return to the starting posture and relax.

EXERCISE 81   Stuttering 2

Starting Posture

Normal Breathing

Lie on the back, legs extended, and feet together.

Bend the elbows 'L' shaped, with the upper arms at the shoulder level. Point the hands in the direction of the head. Make fists.

Relax in this posture briefly, then, inhale.

Extension

Exhaling

Pull the chin in. Stretch the Achilles tendons. Without bending your knees, raise both legs to the ceiling.

Keeping your elbows firmly on the floor, stretch them out to the sides as far as possible.

Inhale deeply, then, retain the breath while holding this posture for a few seconds.

Corrective Movement

Exhaling

Without bending the knees, slowly swing the legs down to the right and then to the left, as far as possible. Stop just short of the floor each time.

(As you move the legs to one side, press down firmly on the floor with the opposite arm)

Inhale, return to the starting posture and relax.

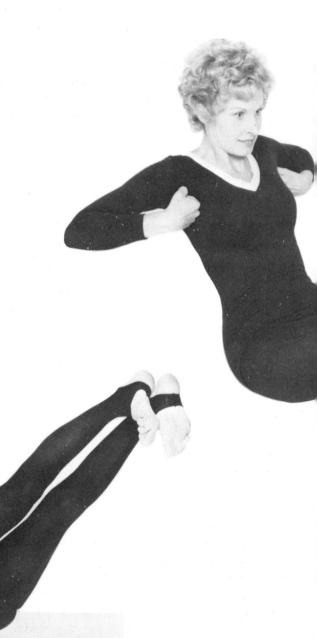

EXERCISE 82 Stuttering 3

Starting Posture
Lie on the back, legs extended, and feet together.

Bend the knees and bring the feet up toward the buttocks.

Make fists and place them under the armpits, letting the elbows rest on the floor.

Relax in this posture briefly, then, inhale.

Extension
Exhaling

Pull the chin in.

Keep your elbows firmly on the floor, stretch out to the sides as far as possible. Press the knees together rightly.

Inhale deeply, then, retain the breath while holding this posture for a few seconds.

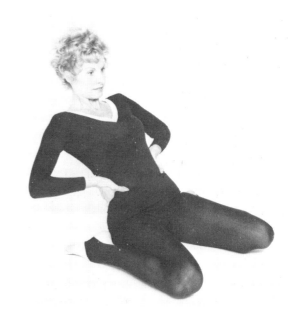

EXERCISE 83 Stuttering 4

Starting Posture
Normal Breathing

Kneel down, back spread straight, knees together, and feet spread waist-width.

Lower the buttocks to the floor and sit between the feet.

Spread the knees apart about waist-width and place the hands on the lower back just above the waist.

Lean back slowly until the head and back are resting on the floor.

Relax in this posture briefly, then, inhale.

Extension
Exhaling

Stretch the elbows down toward the feet, while pushing down on the back firmly with both hands.

Pull the chin in and continue to spread the knees apart.

Inhale deeply, then, retain the breath while holding this posture for a few seconds.

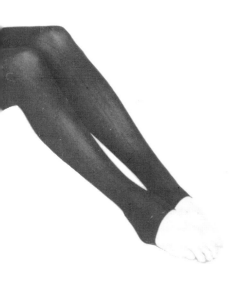

Corrective Movement
Exhaling

Sit up as far as possible, keeping the feet firmly on the floor.

After you finish exhaling, hold this posture and retain the breath for a few seconds. Then, inhale, return to the starting posture and relax.

Corrective Movement
Exhaling

Sit up as far as possible.

After you finish exhaling, hold this posture and retain the breath for a few seconds. Then, inhale, return to the starting posture and relax.

EXERCISE 84 Stuttering 5

Starting Posture

Normal Breathing

Lie on the back, legs extended, and feet spread one and a half times waist-width.

Rest the chin in the hands and rest the elbows on the floor about shoulder-width apart.

Relax in this posture briefly, then, inhale.

Extension

Exhaling

Relax the Achilles tendons.

Stretch the elbows forward.

Inhale deeply, then, retain the breath while holding this posture for a few seconds.

Corrective Movement

Exhaling

Without bending the knees, slowly raise the legs off the floor and spread them apart as far as possible.

At the same time, lift the elbows up off the floor and spread them out as much as possible.

Lift the upper chest off the floor and bring the face parallel to the ceiling.

After you finish exhaling, hold this posture and retain the breath for a few seconds. Then, inhale, return to the starting posture and relax.

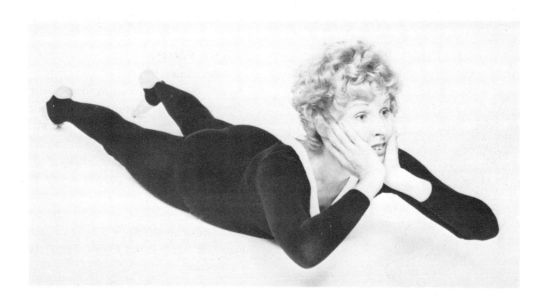

EXERCISE 85 Stuttering 6

Starting Posture

Normal Breathing

Stand with the feet spread about two times waist-width and point the toes outward to a 45 degree angle.

Make fists, placing them under the armpits. Raise the elbows straight upwards without raising the shoulders.

Pull the chin in, straighten the back.

Lower the hips straight down, bending the knees.

In this posture, try to adjust the position of the elbows and knees as follows:

1.) Elbows—they should be extending straight to the sides.

2.) Knees—when you lower the hips, keep the knees spread apart, over the feet (Fig. A).

Relax in this posture briefly, then, inhale.

Extension

Exhaling

Lean the whole body to one side in the following manner:

Keeping the right knee bent in the same position, lift the right leg off the floor as high as possible.

At the same time, extend the right arm straight out to the side.

Keep the face forward and lean as far as possible to the left (Fig. B).

Inhale deeply, then, retain the breath while holding this posture for a few seconds.

Corrective Movement

Exhaling

Exhaling forcefully, return to the starting posture placing the body weight squarely on the right foot as you place it firmly on the floor.

Inhale in the starting posture and repeat the exercise—this time, lifting the left leg and leaning to the right.

Repeat the exercise several times, leaning to both sides. Rest for at least a minute before continuing.

EXERCISE **86** **Stuttering 7**

Starting Posture

Normal Breathing

Stand the toes on a line, feet spread waist-width. Point the feet outwards slightly. Starting with the arms at the sides, raise them straight up behind you, with the palms up. Make fists—thumbs inside (Fig. A).

Relax in this posture briefly, then, inhale.

Extension

Exhaling

Straighten the spine and lower the hips by tightening the anus, and pulling in the chin. Tighten fists and raise the arms up higher. Inhale deeply, then, retain the breath while holding this posture for a few seconds.

Corrective Movement

Exhaling

Do the following movement simultaneously as you exhale forcefully:

HIPS: Suddenly drop the torso down-ward, keeping the spine straight.

ARMS: Keeping the arms straight, swing them downward and forward forcefully, so that they are extended in front of the waist, fists turned inward.

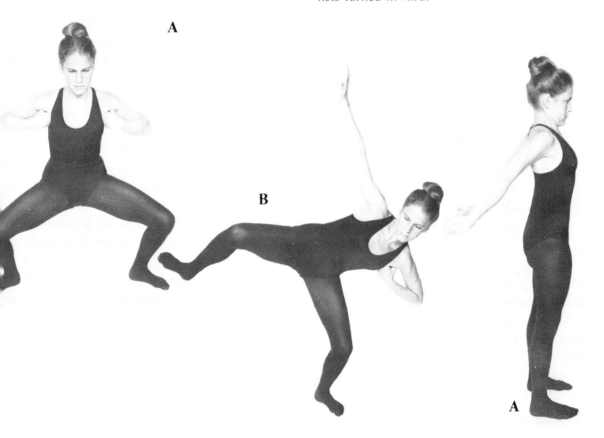

A

B

A

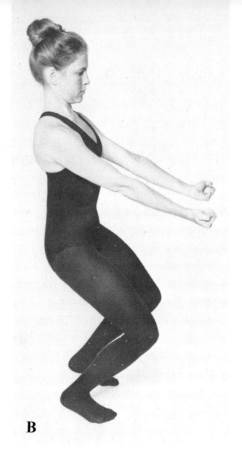

B

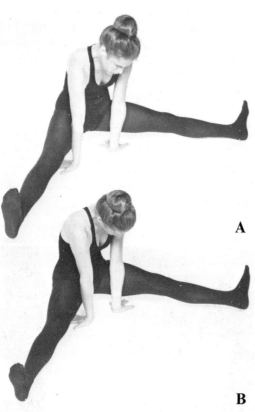

A

B

When you complete this motion, the arms should be almost parallel to the thighs and the weight should be balanced on the balls of the feet (Fig. B). (Keep the chin pulled in firmly as you do this movement.)

After you finish exhaling, hold this posture and retain the breath for a few seconds. Then, inhale, return to the starting posture and rest briefly with the arms at the sides.

EXERCISE **87**   **Stuttering 8**

Starting Posture
Normal Breathing
Sit on the floor, legs extended and feet spread as far as possible.

Place the hands on the floor between the legs, forearms against the inside of the thighs.

(The palms should be down, fingertips pointing back toward the legs (Fig. A).

Relax in this posture briefly, then, inhale.

Extension
Exhaling
Pull the chin in. Stretch the Achilles tendons. Straighten the back and lift the buttocks a few inches off the floor. Inhale deeply, then, retain the breath while holding this posture for a few seconds.

Corrective Movement
Exhaling
Push down on the floor with both hands. Tense the lower abdomen and lift both legs completely off the floor (Fig. B).

At this point you should be supporting yourself only on your hands.

After you finish exhaling, hold this posture and retain the breath for a few seconds. Then, inhale, return to the starting posture and relax.

If you find this exercise too difficult at present, try (1) lifting one leg as a time and (2) leaning the head and torso foward slightly (Fig. B).

Insomnia

Depth of sleep is determined by depth of relaxation of layered brain tissue. In shallow sleep only new brain tissue is relaxed. When old brain tissue relaxes, sleep is deep and little is required.

Since old brain tissue is the activity center for desire, instinct and emotion, a keyed-up emotional state stimulates the brain; therefore, to sleep or relax is difficult. It is important to let go of anxiety or worry before sleeping. Prayer, breathing exercise and zazen are excellent means to peace of mind. However, a truly religious spirit appreciates even not being able to sleep. Such time may be used for study or work rather than begrudged as wasteful sleeplessness. That, then, is joyful acceptance of and obedience to fate given by Kami.

Depth of sleep is also correlative to physiology, as old brain tissue is related to the state of internal organs. For example, a full bladder, stomach or congested intestines adversely stimulate the body so that deep sleep is inhibited. Evacuation and urination before going to sleep are advised.

The new brain tissue must also be relaxed to obtain deep sleep; otherwise, a person finds it difficult to fall asleep and does not enter deep sleep until early in the morning. In order to fall asleep easily, it is necessary to relax the muscles and deepen the breathing, thus putting in order the vagus nerves and stabilizing brain waves. Besides deep breathing, prayer, zazen and laughing gyoho are recommended.

Dis-ease, in general, prevents sound sleep. In such cases, or in any case of insomnia, sleeping pills are not advised. They destroy brain cells, thus impairing thinking ability.

In actuality, excess sleep is more harmful than lack of sleep; excessive amounts numb the nervous system and harden the muscular structure. The insomniac's problem is not that he/she sleeps too little, but that he/she sleeps too shallowly. He/She should discover the dis-ease preventing deep sleep and cooperate with his physiology to heal himself/herself.

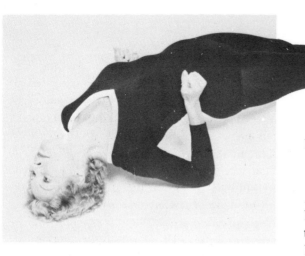

EXERCISE 88   Insomnia 1

Starting Posture
Normal Breathing
Lie on the back, legs extended, and feet together.
Place the arms down at the sides with the palms against the thighs.
Now point the hands straight up toward the ceiling, keeping the elbows on the floor and in close to the chest. Make fists.
Relax in this posture briefly, then, inhale.
Extension
Exhaling
Pressing down on the floor with the elbows, raise up on the top of the head. Point the toes forward. Pull the chin in.
Raise the whole body off the floor as high as possible so that only your heels, elbows and the top of your head are touching the floor.
Inhale deeply, then, retain the breath while holding this posture for a few seconds.
Corrective Movement
Exhaling
Lift the elbows off the floor quickly and relax the whole body. Let the back fall flat on the floor.
With the arms down at the sides, inhale and then remain briefly in this relaxed position, breathing normally—with the palms up, Achilles tendons relaxed, and the chin tilted back.

EXERCISE 89   Insomnia 2

Starting Posture
Normal Breathing
Lie on the back, legs extended and feet together.
Place the hands on the chest and rest the elbows on the floor.
Relax in this posture briefly, then, inhale.
Extension
Exhaling
Pull the chin in, stretch the Achilles tendons, and begin to pull on the chest. Keep the elbows on the floor and stretch them out to the sides.
Inhale deeply, then, retain the breath while holding this posture for a few seconds.
Corrective Movement
Exhaling
Continuing to pull upwards on the chest, raise the whole torso and the legs off the floor simultaneously as high as possible.
(Try to raise both the torso and legs up to a 30 degree angle from the floor, and keep the elbows stretched out to the sides. At this point you should be balancing on the base of the spine.
After you finish exhaling, hold this posture and retain the breath for a few seconds. Then, inhale, return to the starting posture and relax.

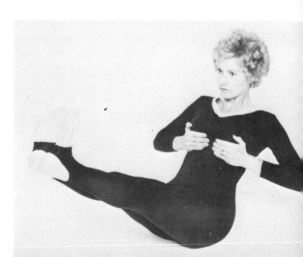

EXERCISE **90**   **Insomnia 3**

Starting Posture
Normal Breathing
Kneel with the back straight and the arms raised straight up overhead.
Bring the feet together, knees spread waist-width apart. Sit down on the feet.
Now slowly lean back until the backs of the hands and the top of the head are resting on the floor.
Relax in this posture briefly, then, inhale.
Extension
Exhaling
Pull the chin in.
Press the knees down on the floor.
Stretch the arms out as far as possible.
Inhale deeply, then, retain the breath while holding this posture for a few seconds.
Corrective Movement
Exhaling
Raise up on the top of the head and arch the back and take the buttocks off the floor as high as possible.
As you arch up in this manner, press down firmly on the floor with the hands, head and knees.
After you finish exhaling, hold this posture and retain the breath for a few seconds. Then, inhale, return to the starting posture and relax.

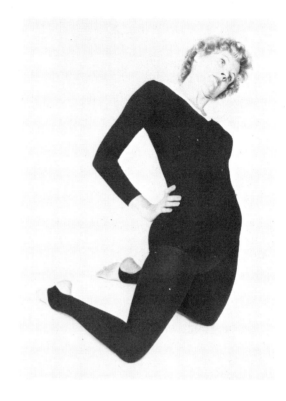

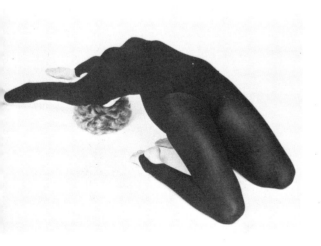

EXERCISE **91**   **Insomnia 4**

Starting Posture
Normal Breathing
Kneel with the back straight and spread the knees and the feet waist-width apart.
Place the hands on the hips.
Stretch the elbows straight back without raising the shoulders.
Relax in this posture briefly, then, inhale.
Extension
Exhaling
Pull the chin in. Lean the shoulders backward and push the hips forward as far as possible.
Inhale deeply, then, retain the breath while holding this posture for a few seconds.
Corrective Movement
Exhaling
Arch the chest back. Bend the neck side to side, ear touching the shoulder while bending the upper torso to the same side.
Inhale, return to the starting posture and relax.

EXERCISE 92   Insomnia 5

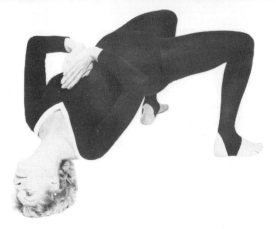

Starting Posture
Normal Breathing

Lie on the back, with legs extended and the feet spread apart one and a half times the waist-width.

Move the feet up toward the hips until the feet are directly below the knees. Keep the feet parallel to each other.

Join the hands together in prayer fashion about three to four inches down from the face. Rest the elbows on the floor.

Relax in this posture briefly, then, inhale.

Extension
Exhaling

Spread the knees apart. Press the hands together, and stretch the elbows out to the sides.

Support on the top of the head, lifting the torso off the floor.

Inhale deeply, then, retain the breath while holding this posture for a few seconds.

Corrective Movement
Exhaling

Without moving the hands and arms, move the torso and legs forward and backward as far as possible with a slow, rocking motion. Inhale, return to the starting posture and relax.

EXERCISE 93   Insomnia 6

Starting Posture
Normal Breathing

Kneel on all fours with the knees and feet together.

Lower the chest and rest the chin on the floor. Extend the arms straight out in front of you with the palms down. The hands are shoulder-width apart.

Relax in this posture briefly, then, inhale.

Extension
Exhaling

Stretch the arms out further, lowering the chest as close to the floor as possible. Raise the hips upwards as much as possible (Fig. A).

Inhale deeply, then, retain the breath while holding this posture for a few seconds.

Corrective Movement
Exhaling

In one smooth motion, arch the chest backward and lift the face up toward the ceiling (Fig. B).

After you finish exhaling, hold this posture and retain the breath for a few seconds.

Then, inhale, return to the starting posture and relax.

A

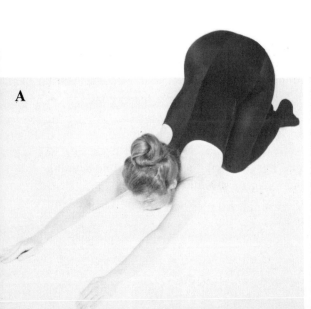

B

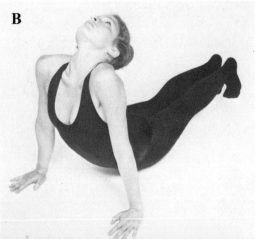

Sexual Difficulties

Sexual potency is determined both psychologically and physiologically. Difficulties such as frigidity, impotence, premature ejaculation and wet-dreams are psychological in origin. Sexual potency is also physiological, related to the operation of the cerebrum, glandular system, sacral and lumbar spinal nerves.

To regulate sexual potency and relieve sexual difficulties, tanden must be strengthened. Deep breathing, particularly emphasizing strength in exhalation and kumbhaka practice provides for sexual endurance. Together, both breathing and tanden control serve to widen the range between tension and relaxation; contraction and expansion of the pelvic area; and movement flexibility.

Sensory awareness is, of course, heightened by matching with an appropriate partner as well as by proper breathing. All the while, it is necessary to keep in mind that love is the foundation element of the spiritual life. Therefore, experimentation with various love-making techniques or work to strengthen the genitals is superficial to healing sexual impotency and other difficulties.

EXERCISE **94** ## Sexual Difficulties 1

Starting Posture
Normal Breathing
Kneel down and sit between the feet. Reach down and grasp the ankles from the outside. Lean back slowly, lie on the back, arms and head on the floor.
Relax in this posture briefly, then, inhale.

Extension
Exhaling
Support on the top of the head and with the elbows, raising the shoulders and chest off the floor.
Inhale deeply, then, retain the breath while holding this posture for a few seconds.

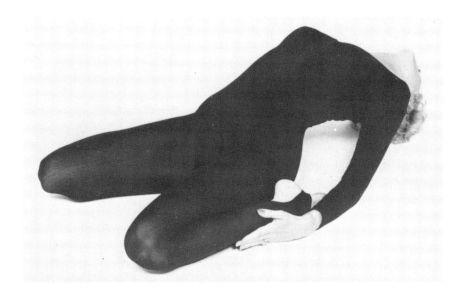

Corrective Movement

Exhaling

Arching the back, slowly bring the knees together, then spread them apart as wide as possible.

As you do this opening and closing movement, press the feet firmly against the hips and keep the knees on the floor.

Inhale, return to the starting posture and relax.

After you finish exhaling, hold this posture and retain the breath for a few seconds. Then, inhale, return to the starting posture and relax.

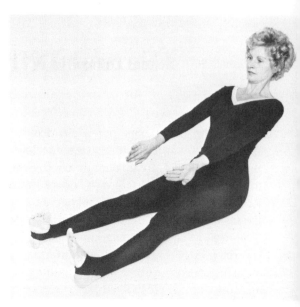

EXERCISE 95 Sexual Difficulties 2

Starting Posture

Lie on the back, legs extended, and feet together.

Turn the feet inward, pressing the toes together, and spread the heels apart.

Place the arms down at the sides with the backs of the hands against the thighs.

Relax in this posture briefly, then, inhale.

Extension

Pressing down on the floor with the elbows, arch the chest upwards, and raise up on the top of the head.

Stretch the Achilles tendons and keep the toes turned inward.

Inhale deeply, then, retain the breath while holding this posture for a few seconds.

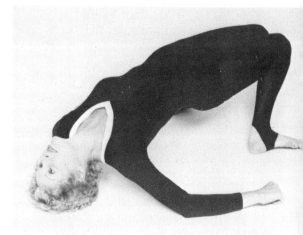

Corrective Movement

Exhaling

Sit up as far as possible, stretching the arms forward.

After you lift the head off the floor, pull the chin in and continue to stretch the Achilles tendons.

After you finish exhaling, hold this posture and retain the breath for a few seconds. Then, inhale, return to the starting posture and relax.

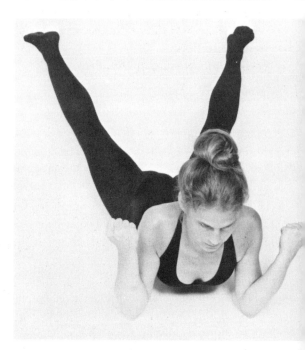

EXERCISE 96   Sexual Difficulties 3

Starting Posture
Normal Breathing
Lie on the back, legs extended, and feet spread waist-width apart.
Bend the elbows 'L' shaped, hands pointing to the feet. Make fists.
Relax in this posture briefly, then, inhale.
Extension
Exhaling
Lift the torso off the floor as high as possible by rising up on the top of the head and pressing down on the floor with the lower arms.
Bring the knees together and raise the hips upwards.
Inhale deeply, then, retain the breath while holding this posture for a few seconds.
Corrective Movement
Exhaling
Rock the whole body forward and backward as far as possible, keeping the knees together. Continue to press down on the floor with the lower arms.
Inhale, return to the starting posture and relax.
Before doing this exercise, loosen the neck by rotating it slowly in both directions as you breathe deeply. Do this for a few minutes until your neck feels loose and flexible.

EXERCISE 97   Sexual Difficulties 4

Starting Posture
Normal Breathing
Lie on the stomach, legs extended, feet together, and forehead on the floor.

Place the elbows on the floor at shoulder level as you raising the head and chest off the floor. Spread the elbows slightly more than shoulder-width.
Point the hands toward the ceiling and turn them so that the palms are facing the feet.
Relax in this posture briefly, then, inhale.
Extension
Exhaling
Pull the chin in. Relax the Achilles tendons. Make fits.
Inhale deeply, then, retain the breath while holding this posture for a few seconds.
Corrective Movement
Exhaling
Raise the legs, opening them slowly as wide as possible. Keep the knees straight.
At the same time, pressing on the elbows to the floor, open the arms down to the side. Move the arms and legs as if to resist an opposing force.

EXERCISE 98   Sexual Difficulties 5

Starting Posture
Normal Breathing
Sit on the floor with the back straight, and legs extended. Spread the feet apart as much as possible.
Make fists and place them under the arm pits.
Relax in this posture briefly, then, inhale.
Extension
Exhaling
Stretch the elbows upwards without lifting the shoulders. Pull the chin in. Stretch the Achilles tendons.
Inhale deeply, then, retain the breath while holding this posture for a few seconds.

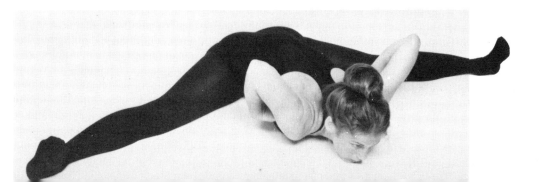

Corrective Movememt

Exhaling

Slowly bend the torso forward as far as possible, trying to touch the chin and chest to the floor. Keep the back and knees straight.

After you finish exhaling, hold this posture and retain the breath for a few seconds. Then, inhale, return to the starting posture and relax.

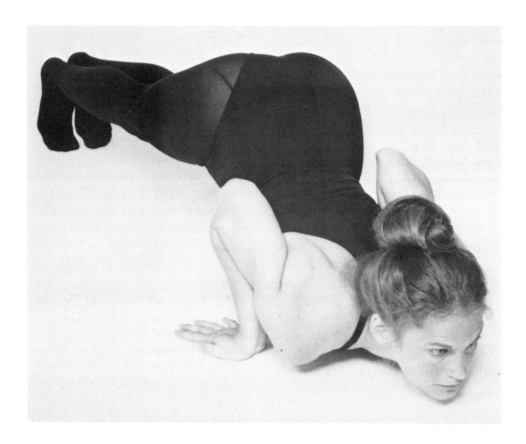

EXERCISE **99** **Sexual Difficulties 6**

Starting Posture

Normal Breathing

Lie on the stomach with legs extended and feet together. Place the chin on the floor. Bend the elbows and put the hands on the floor with the fingers pointing towards the feet.

Relax in this posture briefly, then, inhale.

Extension

Exhaling

Squeeze the elbows in close to the body and

lift the hips off the floor as much as possible. Keep the chin and chest close to the floor. Inhale deeply, then, retain the breath while holding this posture for a few seconds.

Corrective Movement

Exhaling

Slowly push the body forward and backward, supporting yourself only on the hands and toes.

Inhale, return to the starting posture and relax.

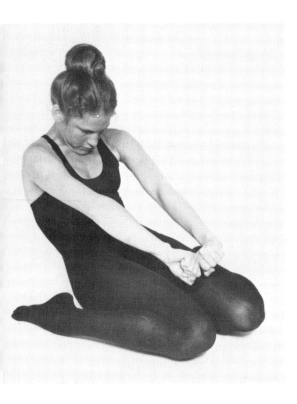

EXERCISE 100 Sexual Difficulties 7

Starting Posture

Normal Breathing

Kneel down and sit between the feet.

Stretch the arms out in front of you at shoulder level, and twist them so that the backs of the hands are touching. Make fists.

Now lean back completely, keeping the arms stretched out at shoulder level.

Relax in this posture briefly, then, inhale.

Extension

Exhaling

Pull the chin in. Stretch the arms forward.

Inhale deeply, then, retain the breath while holding this posture for a few seconds.

Corrective Movement

Exhaling

Sit up, twisting the arms inwards.

(Squeeze the fists together.)

After you finish exhaling, hold this posture and retain the breath for a few seconds. Then, inhale, return to the starting posture and relax.

EXERCISE 101 Sexual Difficulties 8

Starting Posture

Normal Breathing

Sit on the floor, legs extended, and back straight.

Bend the right knee and place the right foot on the left thigh up close to the pelvis.

Place the palms down on the floor, with fingers pointing forward.

Relax in this posture briefly, then, inhale.

Extension

Exhaling

Straighten the back. Pull the chin in. Stretch the Achilles tendon in the extended leg.

Raise the body off the floor supporting yourself only with the hands and left heel.

The right knee should be off the floor, and spread out to the side.

Inhale deeply, then, retain the breath while holding this posture for a few seconds.

Corrective Movement

Exhaling

Continue raising the body off the floor and raise the left heel off the floor as well. After you finish exhaling, hold this posture and retain the breath for a few seconds. Then, inhale, return to the starting posture and relax.

Repeat the same exercise with the left leg on the right thigh. Do the exercise in the posture more difficult.

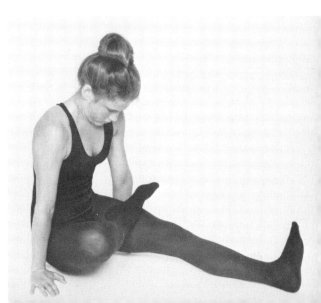

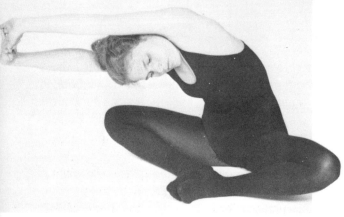

Exercise 102   Sexual Difficulties 9

Starting Posture

Normal Breathing

Sit on the floor. Joining the soles of the feet together, bring the heels up close to the buttocks.

Clasp the hands together, bringing them up toward the ceiling.

Twist the arms so that the palms are facing toward the ceiling.

Relax in this posture briefly, then, inhale.

Extension

Exhaling

Pull the chin in. Stretch the arms upward and press the knees down to the floor.

(In this posture the arms should be pressing against the ears.)

Inhale deeply, then, retain the breath while holding this posture for a few seconds.

Corrective Movement

Exhaling

Slowly bend forward to the center as far as possible, trying to touch the forehead to the floor.

Then inhale, return to the starting posture. Exhaling, bend forward to the left.

Inhale, return to the starting posture. Exhaling, bend forward to the right.

As you bend forward, continue to press the knees down and keep the feet and arms firmly in place.

Note

After each exhalation, retain the breath and posture for a few seconds before inhaling and returning to the starting posture.

Exercise 103   Sexual Difficulties 10

Starting Posture

Normal Breathing

Sit on the floor, legs extended and feet together.

Reach forward and grasp the left ankle with the left hand. Place the right hand on the left knee cap.

Relax in this posture briefly, then, inhale.

Extension

Exhaling

Pull the chin in. Straighten the back.

Stretch the Achilles tendons. Pushing down on the knee cap, straighten the left leg.

Inhale deeply, then, retain the breath while holding this posture for a few seconds.

Corrective Movement

Exhaling

Keeping the back and both legs straight, raise the left leg straight up as you lean the torso forward. Rotate the head so that the left ear touches the left knee.

After you finish exhaling, hold this posture and retain the breath for a few seconds. Then, inhale, return to the starting posture and relax.

Repeat the exercise raising the right leg, and do it in the ratio of three to one on the more difficult side.

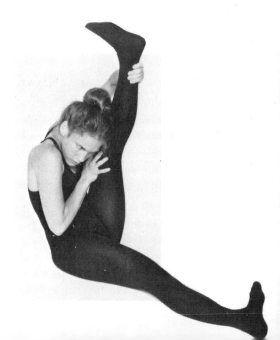

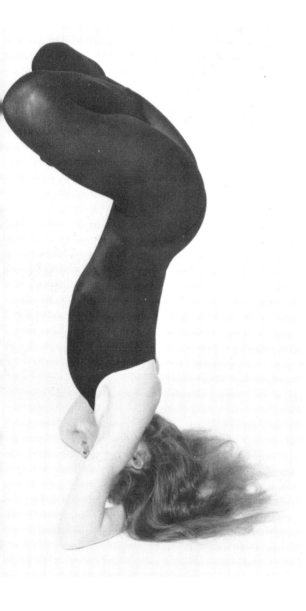

5. Bring the center of gravity toward the head and slowly raise the feet from the floor. Remember never to kick the legs into the air as this defeats the purpose of the pose. Raise the feet slowly with the power of the elbows.

6. Keeping the balance, slowly raise the thighs keeping the knees bent.

7. Extend the Achilles tendons.

Breath Order

Breathe normally in step 1. Inhale in step 2 and move to step 3 while exhaling. Inhale in step 3 and move to step 4 while exhaling. Continue in the same way for the rest of the steps.

Maintain this pose briefly, as you breathe normally.

Extension

Exhaling

Spread the legs apart. Cross them in the full lotus posture, or just put the soles of the feet together, bringing them close to the crotch.

Raise the knees to the ceiling.

Inhale deeply, then, retain the breath while holding this posture for a few seconds.

Corrective Movement

Maintaining this posture, slowly raise and lower the legs as follows.

1) Exhale—lower the legs so that they come close to the abdomen.

2) Inhale—raise the legs in extension.

Repeat this leg movement several times. Then, slowly return to the starting posture, with the legs extended, and relax.

EXERCISE **104** **Sexual Difficulties 11**

Starting Posture

Assume the head stand posture as follows:

1. Place the clasped hands and the elbows on the floor spaced so as to form a triangle. This space should be about the width of the hips.

2. Put the head partly on the hands and partly on the floor.

3. Straighten the knees and raise the hips.

4. Bring the toes toward the head. Keep the knees straight.

EXERCISE **105** **Sexual Difficulties 12**

Starting Posture

Normal Breathing

Lie on the back, knees extended, feet together close to the buttocks.

Extend the arms directly overhead, palms up wards and spread the arms apart slightly wider than the shoulders-width.

Relax in this posture briefly, then, inhale.

Extension
Exhaling

Keeping the feet together, slowly raise the legs and lower straight up off the floor, pointing the toes toward the ceiling.

Press the arms down firmly on the floor.

Corrective Movement
1) Exhale—stretch the Achilles tendons.
2) Inhale—relax the Achilles tendons.

Repeat this simple movement several times. Then inhale as you return to the starting posture and relax.

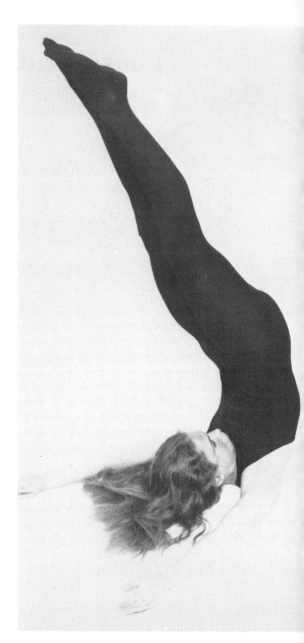

EXERCISE **106**   **Sexual Difficulties 13**

Starting Posture
Normal Breathing

Stand with the feet six inches apart. Then, squat down, spreading the knees apart.

Place the elbows on the inside of the knees, putting the hands on the floor—palms down, fingers forward—a few inches in front of the toes.

Relax in this posture briefly, then, inhale.

Extension
Exhaling

Raise up on the toes as you straighten the back. Pull the chin in.

Lean forward slightly so that the face is parallel to the floor. (At this point the elbows are bent just slightly and pressing firmly against the knees.)

Inhale deeply, then, retain the breath while holding this posture for a few seconds.

Corrective Movement
Exhaling

Raise the toes off the floor, maintaining your balance as you support the whole body on the hands.

After you finish exhaling, hold this posture and retain the breath for a few seconds. Then, inhale, return to the starting posture and relax.

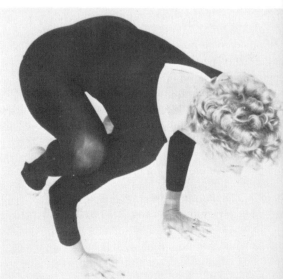

Constipation

Balanced intake and output are essential for healthy life maintenance. Purgation includes vibration, gas, liquid and solid; constipation is the dis-ease of imcomplete purgation of solids.

The problem of constipation is not confined to the colon alone, but is usually only one of a series of related aggravations including diarrhea, general fatigue, dizziness, stiff neck, tight muscles, stomach ache, nauses, thirst, high or low blood pressure and low sexual energy.

Among the causes of constipation not directly related to the function of the large intestine are emotional instability, overacidic stomach, weak-end liver and poor blood circulation in the limbs.

Causes related directly to the large intestine are: weakened intestinal nerves and/or muscles; lack of nutrition absorption; colitis; weakened contractive musculature; and misaligned sacrum and pelvis. The last one, which tends to develop continuous shifting in the position of the intestines, is the most common cause of constipation. Therefore, proper pelvic alignment and strengthening of tanden is necessary for healing. Meanwhile, what a person can immediately undertake to integrate into his/her life is relaxed time and mind to eliminate fully each day; this practice is especially vital for people with hypertension.

Exercise 107 Constipation 1

Starting Posture
Normal Breathing

Assume a full lotus posture or join the soles of the feet, bringing the heels in close to the crotch.

Place the hands—palms down, fingertips forward—on the floor next to the hips. (Keep the arms close to the body.)

Relax in this posture briefly, then, inhale.

Extension
Exhaling

Pull the chin in. Straighten the back, pressing the knees and the hands down to the floor. Lift the buttocks a few inches off the floor, leaning forward slightly.

Inhale deeply, then, retain the breath while holding this posture for a few seconds.

Corrective Movement
Exhaling

Raise the legs completely off the floor. Keeping the back straight, support the entire body with the arms.

After you finish exhaling, hold this posture and retain the breath for a few seconds. Then, inhale, return to the starting posture and relax.

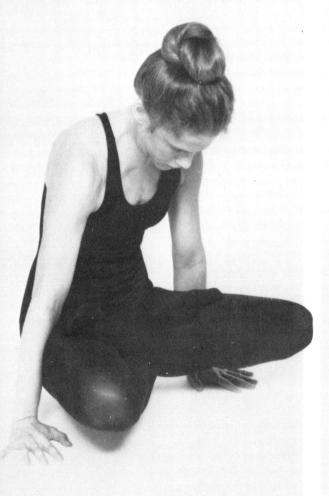

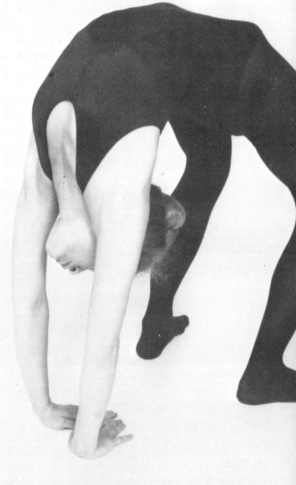

94

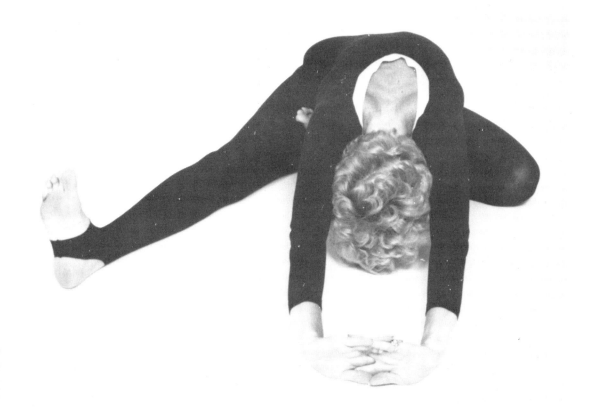

EXERCISE 108 Constipation 2

Starting Posture
Normal Breathing
Lie on the back, legs extended, and feet together. Bring the heels up close to the buttocks.
Bend the elbows, putting the hands on the floor alongside the head, fingertips in the direction of the feet.
Relax in this posture briefly, then, inhale.

Extension
Exhaling
Slowly raise the body off the floor, supporting yourself with the hands, feet, and the top of the head. Then, raise off the head, arching the back upward as high as possible. Thrust the chin out as though you were trying to look at the floor.
Inhale deeply, then, retain the breath while holding this posture for a few seconds.

Corrective Movement
Exhaling
Move the body backwards and forwards with a slow rocking motion, bending the elbows and knees. Keeping the hands and feet firmly in place.
Inhale, return to the starting posture and relax.
Variation on Arch Pose (*Practical Yoga*, p. 32)

EXERCISE 109 Constipation 3

Starting Posture
Normal Breathing
Sit on the floor, the legs extended and feet spread as much as possible.
Now place one foot on top of the opposite thigh, or against the inside of the thigh.
Stretch the arms straight up over the head.
Clasp the hands and twist the arms so that the plams are facing upwards.
Relax in this posture briefly, then, inhale.

95

Extension

Exhaling

Pull the chin in, straighten the back. Stretch the Achilles tendon of the outstretched leg. Now stretch the arms straight up so that the biceps are pressing against the ears. (Keep the arms in this posture throughout the exercise.)

Inhale deeply, then, retain the breath while holding this posture for a few seconds.

Corrective Movement

Exhaling

Bend forward to touch the forehead and chest to the floor, stretching the arms forward. After you finish exhaling, hold this posture and retain the breath for a few seconds. Then, inhale, return to the starting posture and relax.

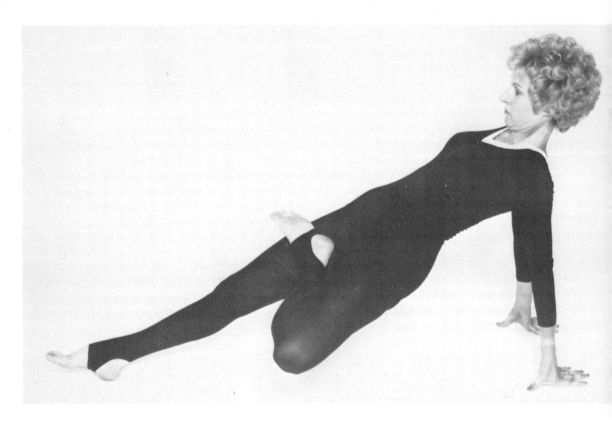

EXERCISE 110 Constipation 4

Starting Posture

Normal Breathing

Sit on the floor, legs extended, and feet together. Place one foot on the opposite thigh or on the inside of the thigh.

Leaning back to a 45 degree angle from the floor, stretch both arms and place the hands on the floor—shoulder-width apart, palms down, fingertips pointing away from the body.

Relax in this posture briefly, then, inhale.

Extension

Exhaling

Pull the chin in. Raise the buttocks off the floor. Stretch the knee out to the side.

Inhale deeply, then, retain the breath while holding this posture for a few seconds.

Corrective Movement

Exhaling

Raise the upper body and hips off the floor as high as possible, supporting yourself with the hands and the heel of the extended leg on the floor.)

Keep the chin down and arch the back up-

ward as much as possible.
After you finish exhaling, hold this posture
and retain the breath for a few seconds.
Then, inhale, return to the starting posture
and relax.

EXERCISE 111   Constipation 5

Starting Posture
Normal Breathing
Kneel with the back straight and spread the
knees waist-width apart.
Place the right arm down at the side. Raise
the left arm up over the head. Twist your left
arm so that the palm is facing inward.
Relax in this posture briefly, then, inhale.

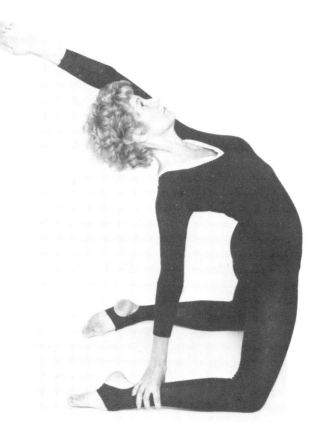

Extension
Exhaling
Pull the chin in. Leaning back, grasp the
right ankle with the right hand. Press the
left arm tightly against the ear.
Inhale deeply, then, retain the breath while
holding this posture for a few seconds.
Corrective Movement
Exhaling
Lean back further. Stretching the left arm
overhead as far as possible, arching the
chest to the ceiling.
After you finish exhaling, hold this posture
and retain the breath for a few seconds. Then,
inhale, return to the starting posture and
relax.
Repeat the exercise, raising the right arm.
Do the exercise more in the posture more
difficult.

EXERCISE 112   Constipation 6

Starting Posture
Normal Breathing
Lie on the back, elbows bent, and hands
under the back. Grasp one wrist with the
other hand. Bend the knees, placing the hips
between the feet.
Relax in this posture briefly, then, inhale.
Extension
Exhaling
Pull the chin in. Press the elbows and knees
down to the floor.
Inhale deeply, then, retain the breath while
holding this posture for a few seconds.
Corrective Movement
Exhaling
Supporting on the top of the head, arch
the back and hips off the floor as high as
possible.
Move the hands up closer to the head.
After you finish exhaling, hold this posture
and retain the breath for a few seconds.
Then, inhale, return to the starting posture
and relax.

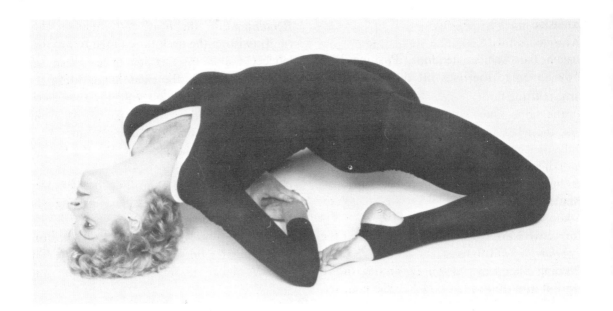

EXERCISE 113 **Constipation 7**

Starting Posture
Normal Breathing

Lie on the stomach, legs extended, forehead on the floor, and feet spread waist-width apart.

Place the hands, palms down next to the shoulders. Arch back as far as possible so that the lower abdomen supports the torso.

Relax in this posture briefly, then, inhale.

Extension
Exhaling

Bend the knees, bringing the feet up close to the head. Arch your head and torso back further until your face is parallel to the ceiling.

Inhale deeply, then, retain the breath while holding this posture for a few seconds.

Corrective Movement
Exhaling

Keeping the hands in place and the arms straight, stretch the head back and the feet forward, trying to touch the toes to the head.

After you finish exhaling, hold this posture and retain the breath for a few seconds. Then, inhale, return to the starting posture and relax.

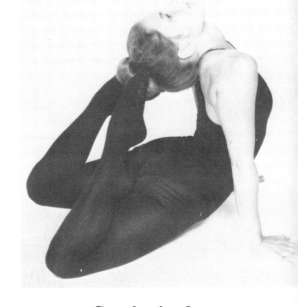

EXERCISE 114 **Constipation 8**

Starting Posture
Normal Breathing

Lie on the stomach, legs extended, and forehead on the floor. Spread the feet apart two times the waist-width.

Place the hands on the floor—palms down, fingertips forward—directly beneath the shoulders.

Relax in this posture briefly, then, inhale.

Extension

Exhaling

Stretch the Achilles tendons. Pushing the body up on to the toes, lift the legs a few inches off the floor.

At the same time, straighten the arms and raise the head and upper body off the floor. Only the hands and toes are touching the floor. The abdomen should be lowered close to the floor but not resting on it.

Inhale deeply, then, retain the breath while holding this posture for a few seconds.

Corrective Movement

Exhaling

Keeping the toes stationary and without bending the elbows or knees, turn the upper body from side to side in the following manner:

Exhaling, turn the head and torso to the right, twisting the neck far enough to see the left heel.

Inhaling, return to the extension position.

Exhaling, turn to the left until the right heel is seen.

Inhaling, return to the extension position.

Do several repetitions of these turning movement. Then, return to the starting posture and rest before doing another set of repetitions.

Gradually increase the number of times you do the excercise. The rate of the breathing must always coincide with the speed of the movements.

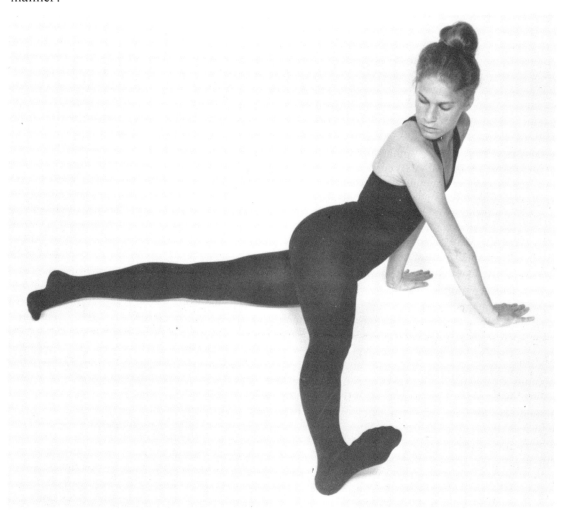

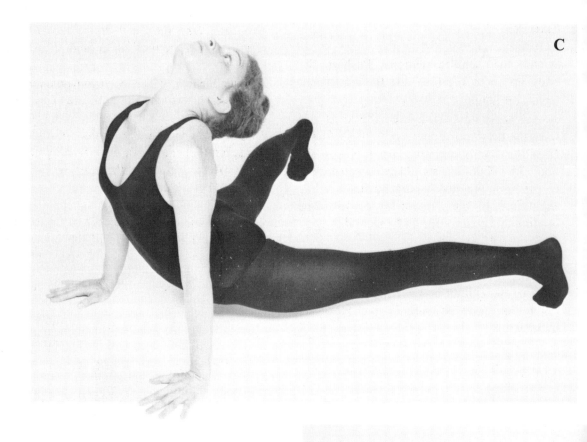

C

EXERCISE 115 Constipation 9

Starting Posture
Normal Breathing
Stand with the legs spread apart two or two and a half times the waist-width. Stretch the arms out in front of you at shoulder level.
Then bend forward, keeping the arms straight. Place the hands on the floor a few feet in front of the toes (Fig. A).
Relax in this posture briefly, then, inhale.

Extension
Exhaling
Stretch the heels backward, and arms forward tucking the head down between the arms, and pulling the chin toward the chest.
At the same time, raise the hips upward as high as possible.
Inhale deeply, then, retain the breath while holding this posture for a few seconds.

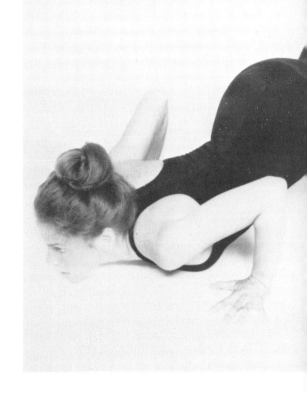

A

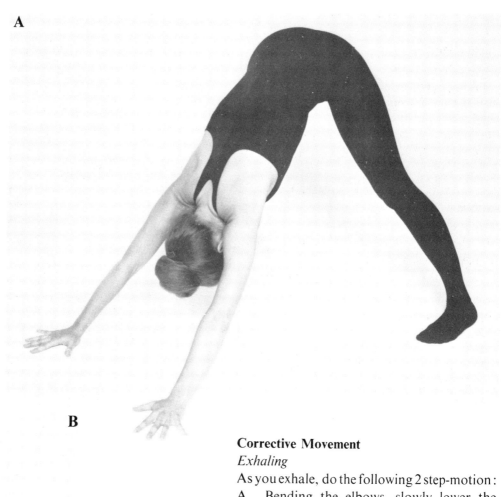

B

Corrective Movement

Exhaling

As you exhale, do the following 2 step-motion:

A. Bending the elbows, slowly lower the chest close to the floor still keeping the hips raised upwards (Fig. B).

B. Now straightening the arms quickly, raise the head and torso upward as much as possible. Thrust the chin upward. (In this position, groin area and legs should be close to the floor, but still not touching the floor. The face should be parallel with the ceiling.) (Fig. C).

Inhaling, return to the extension position.

Do several repetitions of this exercise. Then, rest on the stomach before doing another set of repetitions.

As in the preceeding exercise, gradually increase the speed and number of times you do the exercise. The rate of the breathing must always coincide with the speed of the movements.

EXERCISE 116 Constipation 10

Starting Posture
Normal Breathing

Lie flat on the stomach, legs extended, and forehead on the floor. Spread the feet waist-width.

Bending the knees, bring the feet toward the head. Now reach back and grasp the ankles on the inside.

Relax in this posture briefly, then, inhale.

Extension
Exhaling

Pull the ankles toward the head, arching the back up off the floor (Fig. A).

Inhale deeply, then, retain the breath while holding this posture for a few seconds.

Corrective Movement
Exhaling

Slowly rock the whole body forward and backward as far as possible (Fig. B).

Inhale, return to the starting posture and relax.

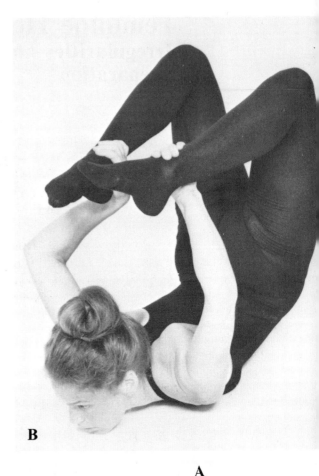

B

A

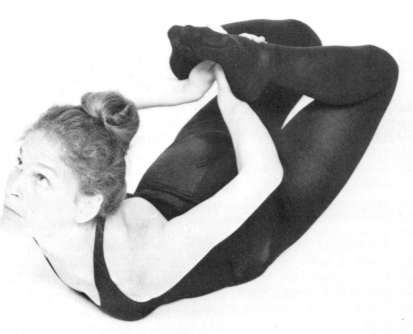

Feminine Health Care: Menstrual Irregularities and Natural Child-birth Preparation

In general, the causes of feminine problems are over-eating; poor purgation of feces, urine and perspiration; postural distortion, especially rotational misalignment; abdominal blood congestion due to weak limbs and tanden; and psychological instability.

Menstruation is nature's function, an aid to women. Usually, for a short time preceeding the period of menstruation, symptoms of change appear: there is weight gain; hypersensitivity in the genital area; and the breasts swell. During this time, many women crave unusual food and feel emotionally irritated and/or sleepy. Whether or not these symptoms should be heeded depends upon the degree of disturbance; if they are bearable without disruption to regular daily living, they may be considered natural.

During pregnancy, Oriental medicine has recognized a "poisoned" period in some women. Water or body fat retention, high blood pressure and protein in the urine are the indications. So long as these symptoms do not lead to other complications, they are negligible. Women who exhibit the "poisoned" state usually have a weak and twisted third lumbar and unbalanced contractive-expansive ability of the sacro-iliac joints. During the "poisoned" state, purgation is especially limited, causing poor blood quality. Proper diet, fasting and tanden breathing are all recommended.

Child bearing is a natural process. Oki sensei has observed natural child birth in Mongolia and India. However, many women in technological societies require hospitalization and anesthesia or other drugs. When drugs are administered, the drowsiness or sleep state of the mother inhibits proper breathing. The oxygen supply to the embryo is then limited, adversely affecting his/her cerebral cortex and, of course, the embryo.

Labor pain is the result of the action of the uterus and utervix opening, with rhythmic, periodic expansion-contraction of the surrounding muscles. When health is properly maintained, labor pain is almost nonexistent, and the time it takes for childbirth relatively shortened. Excessive labor pain results from general physiological misalignment. For example, a twisted pelvis weakens the expansion-contraction action of the sacro-iliac joints, making passage for the embryo difficult. Shusei taiso, aligning the pelvis and lower spine, is especially recommended for feminine difficulties. The strength of the sacro-iliac joints is directly related to the degree of proper breathing; focusing power in tanden while practicing muscular expansion-contraction is advised for assisting childbirth.

In our modern age abortion is prevalent. It is harmful in that it can cause serious tissue damage, and, when tanden is weak, often results in abdominal blood congestion, which complicates the reproductive system.

Fasting and tanden strengthening are very effective healing methods.

Women must also consider their psychological and spiritual states. During child bearing, life attitude is revealed. The more dependent, fearful and passive a woman is, the more painful will it be to bear a child. Pain resides in the mind. The prospective mother needs to trust the wondrous, natural process of her own mind-body and free her mind from anxiety. Daily practice of meiso is recommended.

A

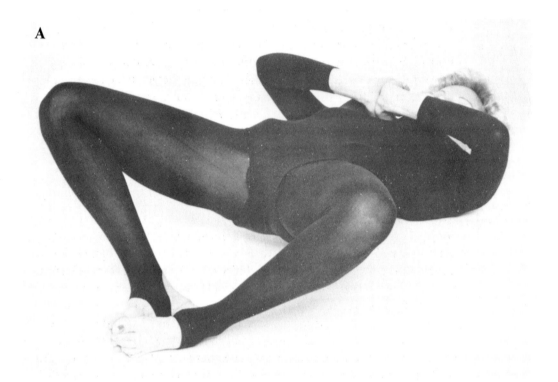

EXERCISE **117**

Feminine Health Care 1

Starting Posture

Normal Breathing

Lying on the back, join the soles of the feet together and bring the heels up close to the buttocks.

Join the hands together above the chest in prayer fashion.

Relax in this posture briefly, then, inhale.

Extension

Exhaling

Pull the chin in. Press the hands together firmly. Spread the knees apart (Fig. A). Raise the hips off the floor.

Inhale deeply, then, retain the breath while holding this posture for a few seconds.

Corrective Movement

Exhaling

Stretch the arms straight out on the floor above the head.

At the same time, stretch the feet downward without dropping the hips (Fig. B).

After you finish exhaling, hold this posture and retain the breath for a few seconds. Then, inhale, return to the starting posture and relax.

B

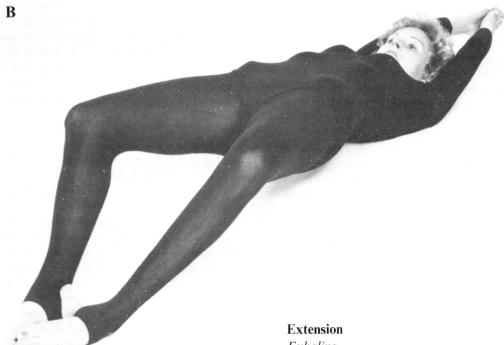

Feminine Health Care 2

Starting Posture
Normal Breathing

Lie the back. Interlock the fingers behind the head just above the neck, elbows resting on the floor.

Cross the legs placing each foot on the opposite thigh in the full lotus posture. (Or, join the soles of your feet together, bringing them close to the buttocks.)

Relax in this posture briefly, then, inhale.

Extension
Exhaling

Pull the chin in. Spread the knees apart, trying to press them down to the floor. At the same time, arch the chest and hips off the floor.

Inhale deeply, then, retain the breath while holding this posture for a few seconds.

Corrective Movement
Exhaling

Slowly bend the upper torso side to side, stretching the opposite side of the chest.

Try to touch the elbow to the knee on the side bent.

Inhale, return to the starting posture and relax.

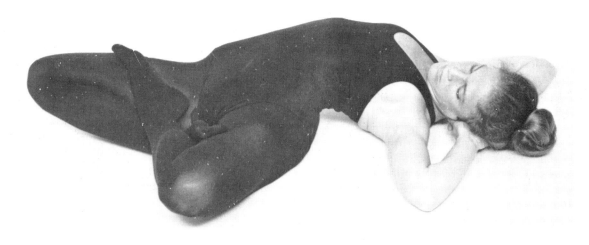

EXERCISE 119

Feminine Health Care 3

Starting Posture
Normal Breathing

Lying on the back, join the soles of the feet together and bring them up close to the buttocks.

Bend the elbows in the 'L' shaped, with the hands pointing to the ceiling. Keep the elbows close to the ribcage. Make fists.

Relax in this posture briefly, then, inhale.

Extension
Exhaling

Press the knees and elbows down toward the floor.

Arch the back off the floor as high as possible.

Inhale deeply, then, retain the breath while holding this posture for a few seconds.

Corrective Movement
Exhaling

Sit up as far as possible, pressing down with elbows (Fig. B).

Inhale, return to the starting posture and relax.

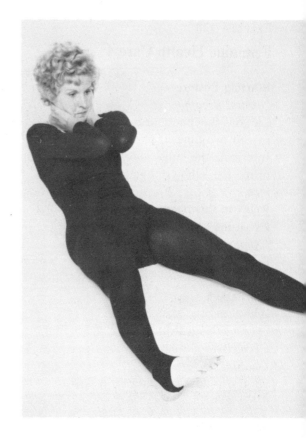

A B

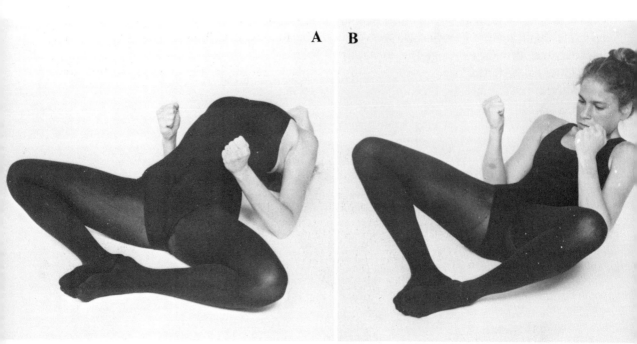

EXERCISE **120**

Feminine Health Care 4

Starting Posture
Normal Breathing

Lie on the back, legs extended, and feet spread two times the waist-width.

Interlock the fingers behind the neck and bring the elbows together in front of the face.

Relax in this posture briefly, then, inhale.

Extension
Exhaling

Pull the chin in. Stretch the Achilles tendons. Turn the toes inward while stretching the heels apart.

Inhale deeply, then, retain the breath while holding this posture for a few seconds.

Corrective Movement
Exhaling

Sit up as far as possible, without bending the knees. Press the elbows together firmly.

After you finish exhaling, hold this posture and retain the breath for a few seconds. Then, inhale, return to the starting posture and relax.

EXERCISE **121**

Feminine Health Care 5

Starting Posture
Normal Breathing

Lie on your stomach.

Bend the right knee and move the right foot in close to the left knee.

Stretch your arms out in front of you at a shoulders with the palms down.

Relax in this posture briefly then inhale.

Extension
Exhaling

Raise your head and chest off the floor pressing down on the floor with the elbows and forearms.

Inhale deeply, then, retain your breath while holding this posture for a few seconds.

Corrective Movement
Exhaling

Raise the left leg off the floor as high as possible without bending the knee.

Press down firmly on the floor with the right knee and the forearms. Lift the face toward the ceiling.

After you finish exhaling, hold this posture and retain the breath for a few seconds. Then, inhale, return to the starting posture and relax.

Repeat this exercise, bending the opposite leg. Do the exercise more in the posture which is more difficult for you.

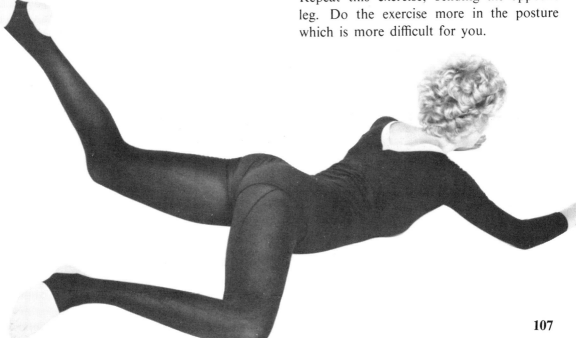

EXERCISE **122**

Feminine Health Care 6

Starting Posture
Normal Breathing
Lying on the back, join the soles of the feet
together and bring the heels up close to
the buttocks.
Place the hands at the bottom of the ribcage.
Rest the elbows on the floor.
Relax in this posture briefly, then, inhale.

Extension
Exhaling
Pull the chin in. Press down on the ribcage
and spread the knees down toward the floor.
Inhale deeply, then retain the breath while
holding this posture for a few sedonds.

Corrective Movement
Exhaling
Sit up as far as possible, pressing down
firmly on the ribcage. Exhale forcefully.
After you finish exhaling, hold this posture
and retain the breath for a few seconds.
Then, inhale, return to the starting posture
and relax.

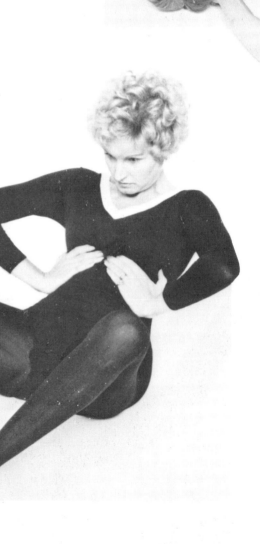

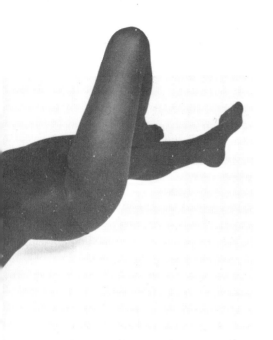

A

Extend the left leg, bending the right knee.
Place your right foot on the left knee.
(Fig. A).
Point the right knee to the ceiling.
Relax in this posture briefly, then, inhale.

Extension

Exhaling

Pull the chin in. Stretch the Achilles tendon
in the left leg (Fig. A).
Keep the elbows on the floor. Stretch them
out to the sides.
Inhale deeply, then, retain the breath while
holding this posture for a few seconds.

Corrective Movement

Exhaling

Raise the hips off the floor as high as possible. (The left knee may bend.) (Fig. B).
This exercise is more effective if you try to
keep the right knee turned down to the
side.
After you finish exhaling, hold this posture
and retain the breath for a few seconds.
Then, inhale, return to the starting posture
and relax.
Repeat the exercise, bending the left knee.
Do the exercise more in the posture which
is more difficult for you.

Exercise 123

Feminine Health Care 7

Starting Posture

Normal Breathing

Lie on the back, fingers interlocked behind
the head just above the neck. Rest the
elbows on the floor.

B

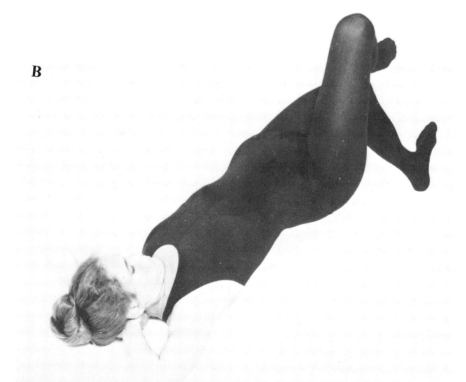

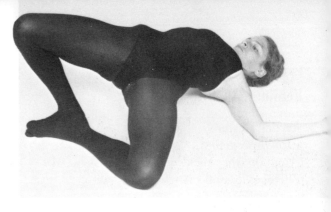

EXERCISE 124
Feminine Health Care 8

Starting Posture
Normal Breathing
Lying on the back, join the soles of the feet together.and bring the heels up close to the buttocks.
Bend the elbows 'L' shape with the fingers pointing in the direction of head. The upper arms are at the shoulder level, palm facing the ceiling.
Relax in this posture briefly, then, inhale.
Extension
Exhaling
Pull the chin in. Keeping the elbows on the floor, stretch, them out to the sides.
Spread the knees apart, stretching the left knee down to the floor.
Inhale deeply, then, retain the breath while holding this posture for a few seconds.
Corrective Movement
Exhaling
Raise the hips off the floor as high as possible while pressing down on the floor with the elbows and the left knee.
After you finish exhaling, hold this posture and retain the breath for a few seconds.
Then, inhale, return to the starting posture and relax.
Repeat the exercise, pressing the right knee down to the floor. Do the exercise more in the posture which is more difficult for you.

EXERCISE 125
Feminine Health Care 9

Starting Posture
Normal Breathing
Lie on the back, legs extended, and feet together. Place the palms underneath the small of the back—about six inches above the waist. Let the elbows rest on the floor.
Relax in this posture briefly, then, inhale.
Extension
Exhaling
Raise the hips off the floor, supporting on the top of the head and elbows.
Stretch the Achilles tendons, and keeping the legs straight.
Inhale deeply, then, retain your breath while holding this posture for a few seconds.
Corrective Movement
Exhaling
Lift one heel about three or four inches off the floor. Without bending the knee, swing the leg slowly out to the side as far as possible.
Inhale as you slowly move the leg back to the center position and lower it to the floor.
Relax briefly in the starting posture.
Repeat the exercise raising the opposite leg. Do the exercise more in the posture which is more difficult for you.

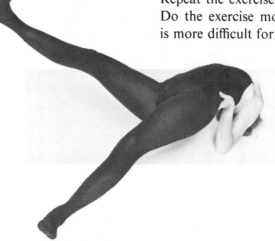

Feminine Health Care 10

Starting Posture
Normal Breathing

Lying on the back, join the soles of the feet together and bring the heels up close to the crotch.

Press the left knee down to the floor. Raise the right knee, and the arms pointing to the ceiling.

Interlock the fingers and twist the arms outwards.

Relax in this posture briefly, then, inhale.

Extension
Exhaling

Pull the chin in. Press the left knee down to the floor. Keep the right leg in place.

Inhale deeply, then, retain the breath while holding this posture for a few seconds.

Corrective Movement
Exhaling

Raise the hips off the floor as high as possible.

After you finish exhaling, hold this posture and retain your breath for a few seconds: Then, inhale, return to the starting posture and relax.

Repeat the exercise with the right knee down to the floor. Do the exercise more in the posture which is more difficult for you.

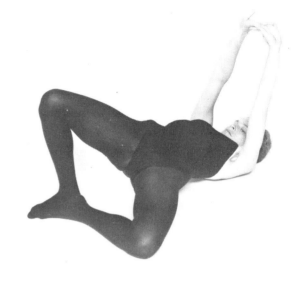

Feminine Health Care 11

Starting Posture
Normal Breathing

Lie on the stomach, feet extended, and forehead on the floor.

Place your hands on the floor—plams down, fingertips forward—beside the shoulders.

Join the soles of the feet together and bring the heels up close to the buttocks.

Relax in this posture briefly, then inhale.

Extension
Exhaling

Squeeze the elbows close to the body and press the feet and knees down firmly and press the feet and knees down firmly on the floor.

Inhale deeply, then, retain the breath while holding this posture for a few seconds.

Corrective Movement
Exhaling

Raise the head and chest off the floor, trying to bring the face parallel to the ceiling. Lift up and back as far as possible without raising the abdomen off the floor.

After you finish exhaling, hold this posture and retain the breath for a few seconds.

Then, inhale, return to the starting posture and relax.

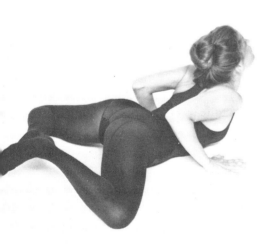

111

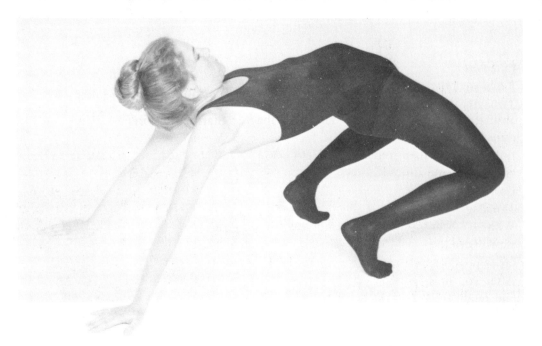

EXERCISE 128

Feminine Health Care 12

Starting Posture

Normal Breathing

Sit on the floor, legs extended, and feet spread waist-width.

Bend the knees bringing the feet close to the buttocks. (The feet should not be directly beneath the knees, but several inches in front of them.)

Lean back to about a 45 degrees angle from the floor and stretch the arms back behind you. Place the hands on the floor slightly more than shoulder-width apart.

Relax in this posture briefly, then, inhale.

Extension

Exhaling

Pull the chin in. Lift the entire body off the floor as high as possible, supporting entirely on the hands and feet.

Inhale deeply, then, retain the breath while holding this posture for a few seconds.

Corrective Movement

Exhaling

Move the body back and forth with a slow rocking motion.

Keep your hips up as high as possible.

Inhale, return to the starting posture and relax.

EXERCISE 129

Feminine Health Care 13

Starting Posture

Normal Breathing

Assume the twist posture as follows:

Sit on the floor, legs extended, and feet spread apart as wide as possible.

Bend the left knee, placing the left heel close to the crotch. Bend the right knee, placing the right foot to the outside of the left knee —the sole of the foot planted firmly on the floor.

Place the right hand on the floor a few inches behind the hips and lean back slightly.

Relax in this posture briefly, then, inhale.

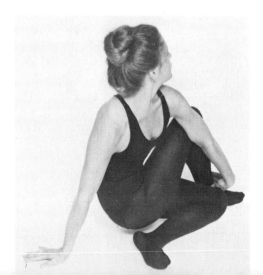

Extension

Exhaling

Twist the torso to the right. With the left arm. Reach down across the outside of the right knee, grasping the right toe.

Inhale deeply, then, retain the breath while holding this posture for a few seconds.

Corrective Movement

Exhaling

Without bending or moving the arms, slowly turn the torso and head to the right as far as possible.

After you finish exhaling, hold this posture and retain the breath for a few seconds.

Then, inhale, return to the extension position and repeat corrective movement.

Repeat the exercise, reversing the positions of your arms and the legs and turning to the left. Do the exercise more in the posture which is more difficult for you.

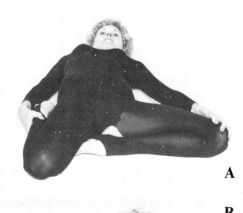

A

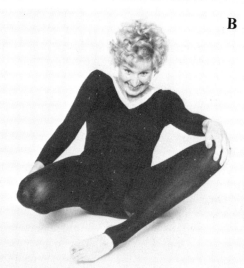

B

EXERCISE **130**

Feminine Health Care 14

Starting Posture

Normal Breathing

Lie on the back, legs extended. Bend the right leg back and place the right foot alongside the right hip. Grasp the right ankle. Place the left foot on the floor against the inside of the right thigh. Place the left hand on the left knee (Fig. A).

Relax in this posture briefly, then, inhale.

Extension

Exhaling

Pull the chin in. Press both knees down to the floor. Arch the back off the floor, resting on the shoulder blades and head.

Inhale deeply, then, retain the breath while holding this posture for a few seconds.

Corrective Movement

Exhaling

Pulling firmly on the knee and ankle, sit up as far as possible (Fig. B).

At the same time, keep the chin pulled in and the back arched upwards.

After you finish exhaling, hold this posture and retain the breath for a few seconds.

Then, inhale, return to the starting posture and relax.

Repeat the exercise, reversing the positions of the legs. Do the exercise more in the posture which is more difficult for you.

EXERCISE **131**

Feminine Health Care 15

Starting Posture

Normal Breathing

Kneel on all fours with the knees and feet together. Place the hands on the floor —fingertips pointing forward—directly beneath the shoulders.

Place the right hand on the back of the neck (Fig. A).

Relax in this posture briefly, then, inhale.

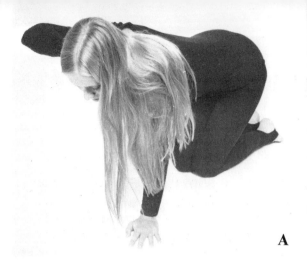

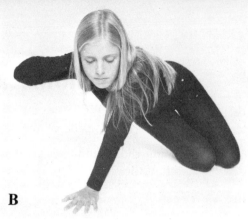

B

A

Feminine Health Care 16

Extension

Exhaling

Press the knees together firmly.

Raise the right elbow. Lift the chin, keeping the back extended.

Inhale deeply, then, retain the breath while holding this posture for a few seconds.

Corrective Movement

Exhaling

Slowly twist the hips down to one side and to the other side as far as possible (Fig. B).

After you finish exhaling, hold this posture and retain the breath for a few seconds. Then, inhale, returning to the starting posture. Lower the hips to the opposite side, exhaling.

Repeat the exercise with the left hand at the side of the head. Do the exercise more in the posture which is more difficult for you.

Starting Posture

Normal Breathing

Lie on the back, legs extended, and feet together. Place the right foot aganist the inside of the left knee.

Place the right hand on the right knee. Place the left hand behind the head just above the neck.

Relax in this posture briefly, then, inhale.

Extension

Exhaling

Pull the chin in. Stretch the right elbow out to the side.

Stretch the Achilles tendon in the left leg.

Inhale deeply, then, retain the breath while holding this posture for a few seconds.

Corrective Movement

Exhaling

Pulling on the right knee and keeping the left elbow stretched upwards, sit up as far as possible.

After you finish exhaling, hold this posture and retain the breath for a few seconds. Then, inhale, return to the starting posture and relax.

Repeat the exercise reversing the position of the legs. Do the exercise more in the posture which is more difficult for you.

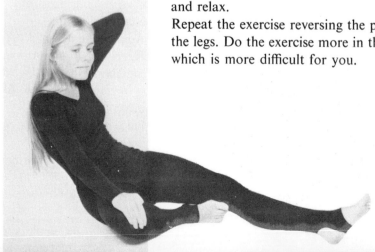

Homorrhoids and Piles

Hemorrhoids and piles are dis-eases not just of the rectum and anal canal, but of the entire body. Hemorrhoids may derive from blood congestion in the veins of the colon, resulting from, for example, pregnancy difficulty, constipation, fallen internal organs, weak legs, mucus accumulated in the intestines, inappropriate drinking and/or smoking, and prolonged sitting. There may also be poor blood circulation in the veins of the rectum and anal canal, resulting from abnormal functioning of the liver and spleen. Yet another possibility is a weakened or inactive sphincter muscle.

Usually pain and bleeding accompanies the inflammation. If there is bleeding without pain, the condition may be canecr of the colon. In such a case, a physical check-up is recommended.

Piles—fissure of the anus—indicated by bursting of the small blood vessels near the anal canal, come from strain due to a condition in which the sphincter is tense and the stool hard. More indirectly, blood congestion in the rectum, poor blood circulation in the legs and constipation cause piles.

Postural distortions observed by Oki Sensei for those with hemorrhoids and piles are similar to those with constipation: the back is rounded; upper thoracic and cervical vertebrae are tight; and the lumbar inflexible. Inevitably, tanden is weak.

EXERCISE **133**   **Hemorrhoids 1**

Starting Posture
Normal Breathing
Stand with the back straight and feet spread
waist-width apart.
Raise the arms directly over head. Clasp the
hands and turn the palms upwards.
Now place the right foot against the inside
of the left thigh.
Relax in this posture briefly, then, inhale.
Extension
Exhaling
Pull the chin in. Stretch the arms upwards.
Place the weight on the inside of the left leg
by pressing the big toe down firmly on the
floor. Spread the right knee outwards.
   Inhale deeply, then, retain while breath
while holding this posture for a few seconds.
Corrective Movement
Exhaling
Keeping the back straight and bending the
left knee and slowly lower the hips straight
down as far as possible.
Inhale, return to the starting posture and
relax.
Repeat the exercise, bending the left knee.
Do the exercise more in the more difficult
posture.

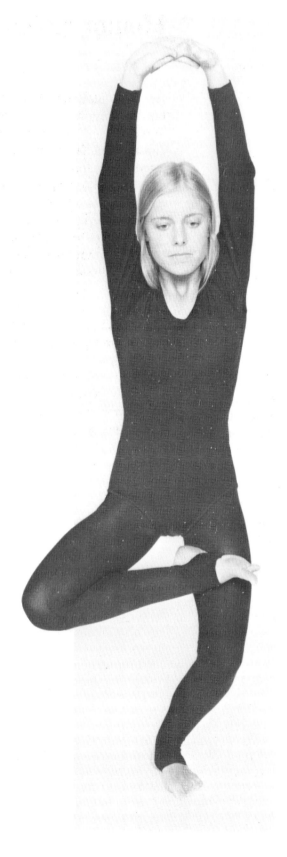

EXERCISE **134**   **Hemorrhoids 2**

Starting Posture
Normal Breathing
Sit, hips between the bent legs.
Raise the arms directly overhead. Clasp the
hand and turn the palms of the hands to the
ceiling.
Now slowly lean back as far as possible,
trying to rest the top of the head on the
floor (Fig. A).
Relax in this posture briefly, then, inhale.
Extension
Exhaling
Press the knees together. Stretch the arms

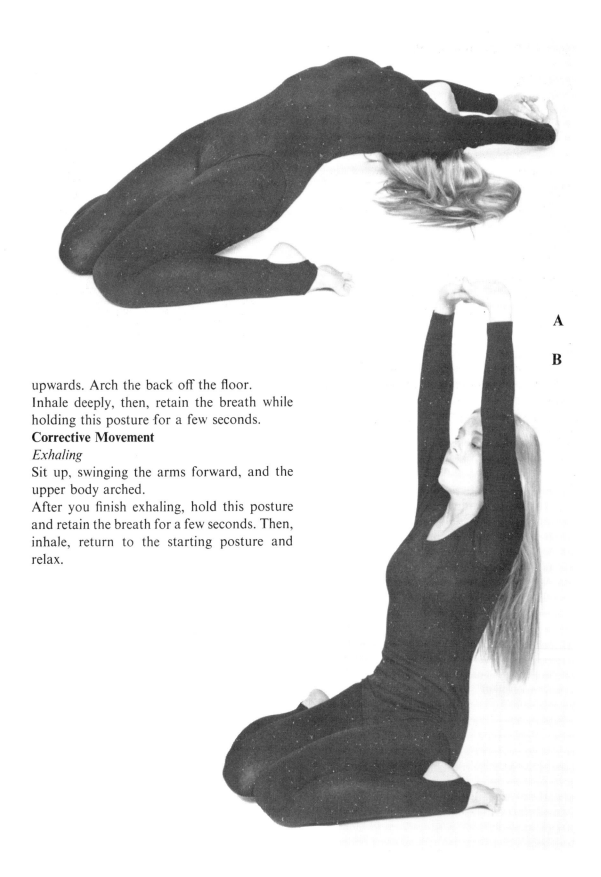

A

B

upwards. Arch the back off the floor.

Inhale deeply, then, retain the breath while holding this posture for a few seconds.

Corrective Movement

Exhaling

Sit up, swinging the arms forward, and the upper body arched.

After you finish exhaling, hold this posture and retain the breath for a few seconds. Then, inhale, return to the starting posture and relax.

EXERCISE 135 Hemorrhoids 3

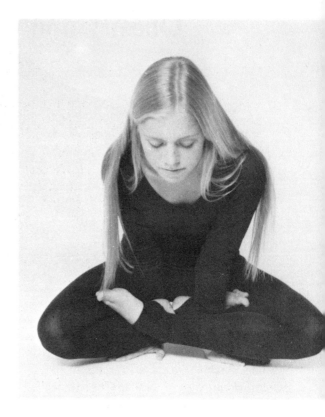

Starting Posture

Normal Breathing

Assume the full lotus posture, or join the soles of the feet together. Place the hands on the floor (palms down, fingertips pointing outward) in the space between the ankles.

Relax in this posture briefly, then, inhale.

Extension

Exhaling

Pull the chin in, straighten the back. Press the hands down to the floor.

Inhale deeply, then, retain the breath while holding this posture for a few seconds.

Corrective Movement

Exhaling

Lift the whole body off the floor.

Hold this posture for several seconds, exhaling slowly.

Inhale, return to the starting posture and relax.

Obesity and Over-weight

Obesity and overweight are related to dietary habits, amount of exercise and psychological state. Overweight indicates an unblanced state, a break-down in proper nutrition absorption. There are three types of excessive retention leading to obesity—water, fat and toxic deposits.

Common to obesity and overweight is an expanded pelvic structure due to tightened sacro-iliac joints. The gyoho, therefore, are designed to correct this distortion. Blood congestion in the abdomen is also common in overweight, as well as accumulation of deep body fat. Therefore, breathing exercise is necessary. All types of overweight contribute to weakening of tanden; the gyoho likewise serves to strengthen tanden.

EXERCISE **136** **Obesity 1**

Starting Posture

Normal Breathing

Lie on the back, legs extended and feet spread apart two times waist-width.

Turn the toes inward and spread the heels out to the sides.

Clasp the hands behind the neck and rest the elbows on the floor.

Relax in this posture briefly, then, inhale.

Extension

Exhaling

Pull the chin in. Bring the elbows together above the chest. Stretch the Achilles tendons.

Inhale deeply, then, retain the breath while holding this posture for a few seconds.

Corrective Movement

Exhaling

Sit up with the elbows together firmly, pulling the head forward.

Continue to stretch the Achilles tendons and avoid bending the knees as you sit up in this manner.

Hold this posture and retain the breath for a few seconds. Then, inhale, return to the starting posture and relax.

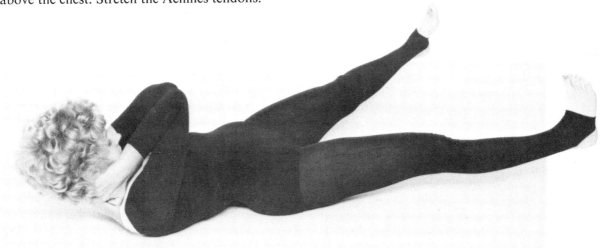

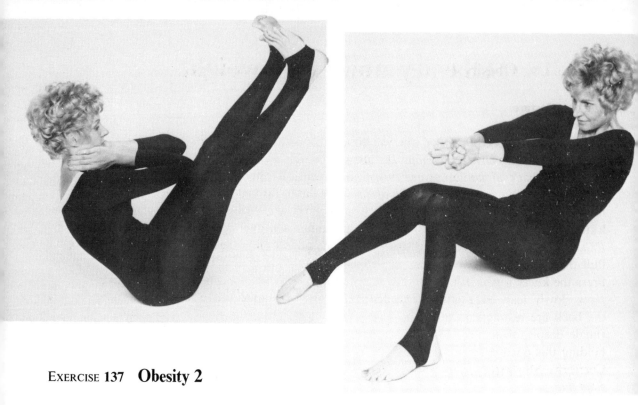

Exercise 137   **Obesity 2**

Starting Posture

Normal Breathing

Lie on the back, legs extended, and feet together.

Turn the feet inward, pressing the toes together, spread your heels apart.

Clasp the hands behind the neck and rest the elbows on the floor.

Relax in this posture briefly, then, inhale.

Extension

Exhaling

Pull the chin in. Bring the elbows together above the chest. Stretch the Achilles tendons. Inhale deeply, then, retain the breath while holding this posture for a few seconds.

Corrective Movement

Exhaling

Pressing the elbows together firmly, and keeping the legs straight, raise the torso and the legs off the floor simultaneously and as high as possible.

While doing this movement, continue to pull firmly on the neck and to stretch the heels out to the sides.

Hold this posture and retain the breath for a few seconds. Then, inhale, return to the starting posture and relax.

Exercise 138   **Obesity 3**

Starting Posture

Normal Breathing

Lie on the back. Bending the knees, bring the feet up close to your buttocks.

Bring the knees together and spread the feet waist-width apart.

Relax in this posture briefly, then, inhale.

Extension

Exhaling

Pull the chin in. Stretch the arms upwards. Press the knees together firmly.

Inhale deeply, then, retain the breath while holding this posture for a few seconds.

Corrective Movement

Exhaling

Sit up as far as possible, stretching the arms forward beyong the knees.

Hold this posture and retain the breath for a few seconds. Then, inhale, return to the starting posture and relax.

120

EXERCISE **139** **Obesity 4**

Starting Posture
Normal Breathing
Sit between the heels.
Stretch the arms overhead, turning the arms
so that the back of the hands are touching.
Make fists.
Relax in this posture briefly, then, inhale.

Extension
Exhaling
Pull the chin in. Stretch the arms upwards.
Press the knees together.
Now slowly lean back until the head and
the back are resting on the floor.
Inhale deeply, then, retain the breath while
holding this posture for a few seconds.

Corrective Movement
Exhaling
Stretching the arms forward, raise the torso
upward.
Hold this posture and retain the breath for
a few seconds. Then, inhale, return to the
starting posture and relax.
Variation on Tanden Strengthening Pose
No. 4 (*Practical Yoga*, p. 50)

A

B

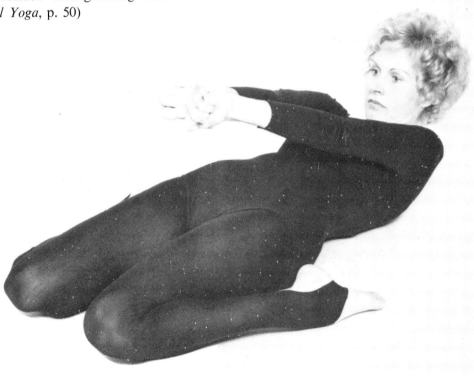

EXERCISE 140   Obesity 5

Starting Posture

Normal Breathing

Lie on the stomach, legs extended, and forehead on the floor. Spread the feet waist-width apart.

Clasp the hands behind, resting the hands on the small of the back.

Relax in this posture briefly, then, inhale.

Extension

Exhaling

Raise the arms upward toward the head as far as possible. Lifting the face toward the ceiling, raise the chest off the floor. At the same time, spread the legs apart and raise the feet off the floor as high as possible without bending the knees.

Inhale deeply, then, retain the breath while holding this posture for a few seconds.

Corrective Movement

Exhaling

Slowly move the whole body back and forth with a slow rocking motion.

Also slowly swing the upper body side to side. Inhale, return to the starting posture and relax.

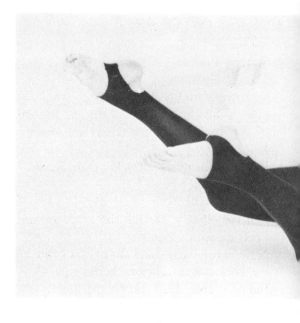

EXERCISE 141   Obesity 6

Starting Posture

Normal Breathing

Sit on the floor. Cross the legs, placing each foot on the opposite thigh in the full lotus posture, or join the soles of the feet together.

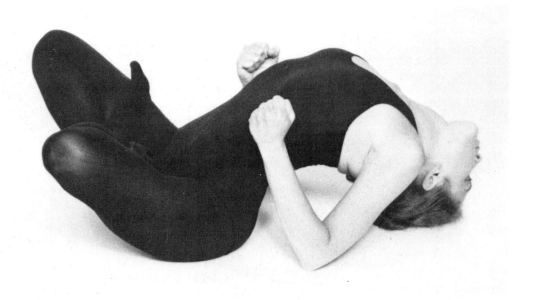

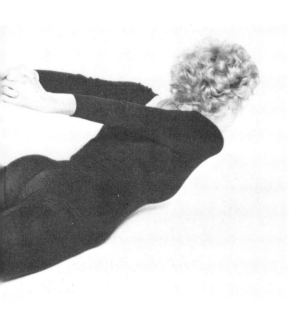

Extension

Exhaling

Pressing the elbows down firmly on the floor, arch the back off the floor as high as possible. Support on the top of the head.

Inhale deeply, then, retain the breath while holding this posture for a few seconds.

Corrective Movement

Exhaling

Keeping the knees spread apart, move the legs up and down—trying to touch the knees to the chest as you lift the legs.

As you move the legs, keep the upper back arched as much as possible and remain on the top of the head.

Inhale, relax into the starting posture.

Holding this posture, lean back completely until the head and the back are resting on the floor. Bring the arms in close to the body.

Bend the elbows so that the hands are pointing straight up at the ceiling. Make fists. Relax in this posture briefly, then, inhale.

EXERCISE 142 Obesity 7

Starting Posture

Normal Breathing

As in the preceding exercise, sit on the floor in the lotus pusture (or with the soles of the feet joined together) and lean back until the head and the back rest on the floor.

Place the hands at the bottom of the shoulder blades.

Relax in this posture briefly, then, inhale.

Extension

Exhaling

Raise the legs and torso straight up off the floor, supporting with the elbows.

Inhale deeply, then, retain the breath while holding this posture for a few seconds.

Corrective Movement

Exhaling

Spread the knees out to the sides.

Keeping the head in place, turn the legs and hips from left to right as far as possible with a slow twisting motion.

The back should be perpendicular to the floor while the legs should remain off the floor.

Inhale, return to the starting posture and relax.

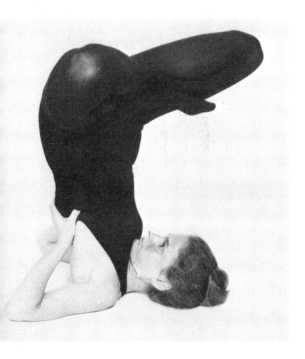

EXERCISE 143 Obesity 8

Starting Posture
Normal Breathing
Kneel with knees and feet together. Support the chin with the heels of the hands.
Place the elbows close to the chest.
Relax in this posture briefly, then, inhale.

Extension
Exhaling
Raising the elbows up to shoulder level, begin pushing the head back while still keeping the back straight.
Inhale deeply, then, retain the breath while holding this posture for a few seconds.

Corrective Movement
Exhaling
Leaning back as far as possible, pushing the chin back until the elbows are pointing directly up toward the ceiling.
At the same time, extend the pelvis forward as far as possible.
Hold this posture and retain the breath for a few seconds. Then, inhale, return to the starting posture and relax.

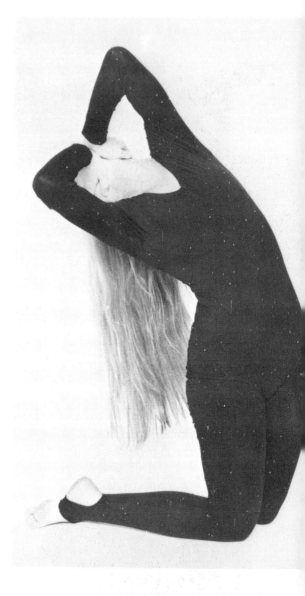

EXERCISE 144 Obesity 9

Starting Posture
Normal Breathing
Stand with the back straight and spread the feet apart two times the waist-width.
Keep the feet parallel.
Extend the arms behind you at about shoulder level. Clasp the hands.
Relax in this posture briefly, then, inhale.

Extension
Exhaling
Raise the arms upward without bending the elbows. Press the hands together firmly.
Drop the hips straight down, keeping the back straight. Avoid bending forward. Press the knees together firmly.
Inhale deeply, then, retain the breath while holding this posture for a few seconds.

Corrective Movement
Exhaling
Swing the arms from left to right as far as you can, keeping your back straight and the face, forward.
Continue pressing the knees together while doing this movement.
Inhale, return to the starting posture and relax.

124

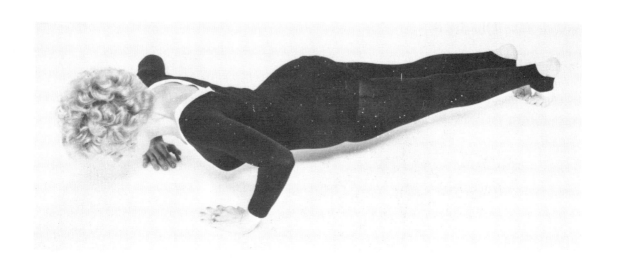

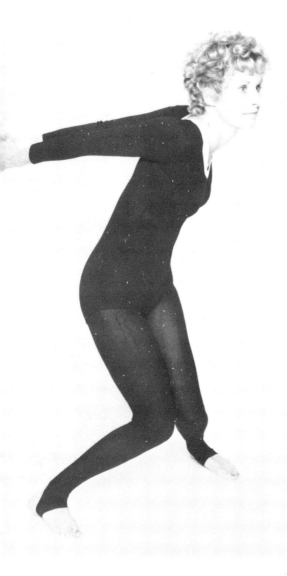

EXERCISE 145 Obesity 10

Starting Posture

Normal Breathing

Lie on the stomach, legs extended, feet together, and forehead on the floor.

Place the hands on the floor (fingertips pointing in toward the chest) a few inches away from the shoulders.

Relax in this posture briefly, then, inhale.

Extension

Exhaling

Keeping the toes in place, spread the heels apart as much as possible.

At the same time, keeping the hands in place, move the elbows up to shoulder level.

Inhale deeply, then, retain the breath while holding this posture for a few seconds.

Corrective Movement

Exhaling

Keeping the chin pulled in, slowly do several push-ups. Raise the body off the floor only a few inches so that the chest rises just above the level of the elbows. (As you lower the body, avoid touching the floor.)

Continue this movement until you finish exhaling).

Inhale, return to the starting posture and relax.

125

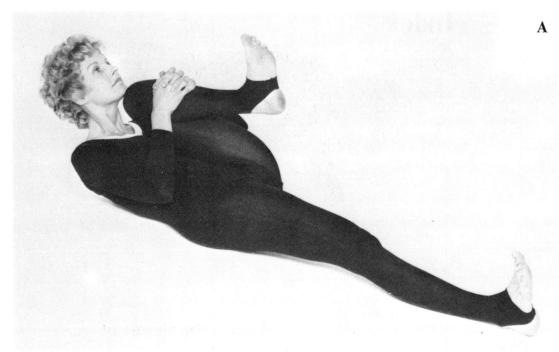

EXERCISE 146 Obesity 11

Starting Posture
Normal Breathing

Lie on the back, legs extended, and feet together.

Clasp the hands around one knee and pull the knee up toward the chest (Fig. A).

Relax in this posture briefly, then, inhale.

Extension
Exhaling

Stretch the Achilles tendons. Pull the knee tightly against the chest.

Pull the chin in. Lift the head off the floor. Inhale deeply, then, retain the breath while holding this posture for a few seconds.

Corrective Movement
Exhaling

Sit up, pulling the knee against the chest. Hold this posture and retain the breath for a few seconds. Then, inhale, return to the starting posture and relax.

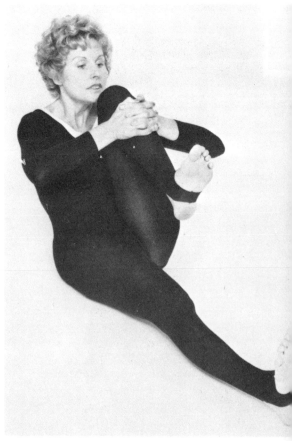

126

Index

shiatsu 9
Shusei Gyoho 9, **10**, 11
Shusei Taiso 6, 9, 12, 13, 15, **17**, 55, 103
sinus **55**
snor **71**
spinal misalignment 17
spinal stimulation **17**
stiff neck 93
stiff shoulders 49
stomach ache 93
stomach, fallen **49**
stuffy nose 55
stutter **75**

taiso 9, 11
Taoism 10
thirst 93

tight muscles 93

Undo 9

Western medicine 9, 10, 11, 12
Western society 5, 9
Westerners throughout 9
wholistic healing 11

Yang 10, 14 ,17
Yin 10, 14, 17
Yoga 9, 10
yosetsu 17

zazen 59, 81